Great Expectations

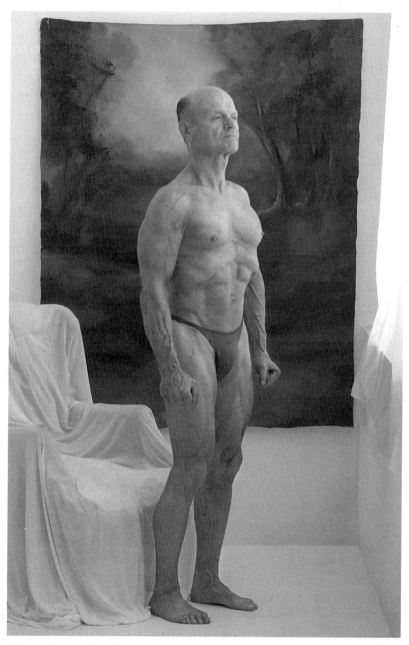

The author at 70. *Photo by Laszlo Bencze in Pat Berrett's natural-light studio*

Great Expectations

Health
Fitness
Leanness
Without Suffering

by Clarence Bass

Clarence Bass' **RIPPED**™ Enterprises
Albuquerque, New Mexico

ISBN 978-0-9747682-4-3

Published by Clarence Bass' Ripped Enterprises
P.O Box 51236
Albuquerque, New Mexico 87181 U.S.A.
505-266-5858 FAX 1-505-266-9123
E-mail: cncbass@aol.com
Web Site: www.cbass.com

RIPPED ™ is the trademark of Clarence and Carol Bass

Library of Congress Control Number: 2007908091

ISBN: 978-0-9747682-4-3

Covers designed by Randy McMullen, Visual Communications
Albuquerque, New Mexico

Composition by Wright Graphics
Albuquerque, New Mexico

Manufactured by Thomson-Shore, Inc.
Dexter, Michigan, U.S.A.

Photos on front cover and back cover by *Laszlo Bencze*

Dedication

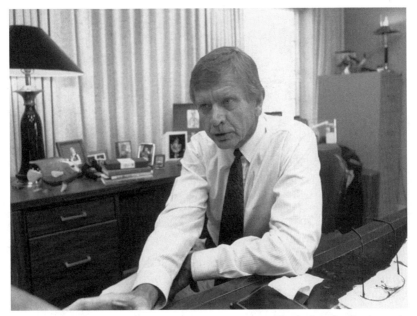

Photo by Justin Joseph

To Arnie Jensen, M.D., who introduced me to the Cooper Clinic, the world leader in preventive medicine, and became my friend. He practices what he preaches, and has the highest expectations for his patients and himself.

WARNING

Any application of the recommendations in this book is at the reader's sole discretion and risk.

The information in this book is intended for people in good health. If you have medical problems—of any nature—see your doctor before starting a diet or exercise program. Furthermore, even if you have no known health problems, it is advisable to consult your doctor before making any major changes in your lifestyle.

Invariably, if you are out of shape and want to start training, follow the advice of the American Medical Association: "Start slowly and increase the vigor and duration of the activity as your fitness improves."

CONTENTS

"The human brain is a magical biocomputer. It sends us energy when we send it something clearly and logically inspiring."

Steve Chandler
Reinventing Yourself

"How you think is everything."

Investors Business Daily

Chapter One

Great Expectations

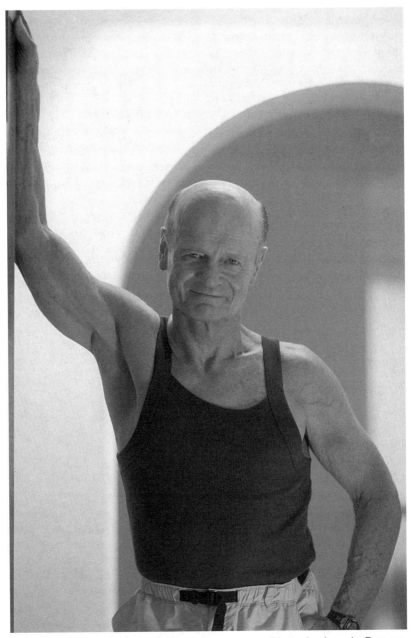

Attitude Matters

My expectations are great, and I want to share that vision with you.

As I begin writing this book, I'm six weeks past my 69th birthday and four days away from the first photo session in my 70th year. In the four years since my last photos, I've had two major surgeries—after going my entire adult life without spending one night in the hospital. Nevertheless, I expect the photos to be as good as before, in some ways perhaps better.

Why not? My condition was good at 60 and 65 (also 30, 40 and 50); and I expect it to be good at 70. That's contrary to general expectations, I know, but working to improve my fitness and physique at 60 and 65 also went against the tide. My workouts are going well. I see little or no change when I step on my Tanita Body Composition Monitor or when I look in the mirror. Why should I expect anything different now? My approach is to work hard, continue to challenge myself—and expect the best. As Dr. Michael F. Roizen wrote in *The Real Age Makeover* (2004, HarperCollins): "A positive attitude really does make a difference."

Whether you are young or old, expect—and work for—the best. If you think you can, you probably can. That's the basic theme of this book, that's what it's about.

I'm going to tell you things I've learned and experienced that will help you live up to your own *great expectations.*

Expectation and Action

High or low expectations have a major impact on your results. I know because I've lived it. But you don't have to take my word for it. Science supports what I am telling you. A study reported in the *Journal of General Internal Medicine* (October 2005) found that expectation and action are closely related. (The study deals with people over 65, but my experience tells me that it has general application.)

The study surveyed 636 older adults regarding their age expectations (low to high) and their physical activity in the previous week.

They found that participants who expect their health to decline were much less likely to be physically active compared to those who had high expectations.

"Harboring low age-expectations may act as a barrier to physical activity among sedentary older adults," lead author Dr. Catherine A. Sarkisian and her colleagues concluded. Low expectations are likely to be a self-fulfilling prophesy.

4

As my friend Dr. Waneen Spirduso and her co-authors wrote in *Physical Dimensions of Aging* (Human Kinetics, Second Edition, 2005), "A vicious cycle develops. As people age, they become less active. The less active they are, the less physical ability and endurance they have. The less physical ability they have, the less inclined they are to be physically active. And the less active they are, the more physical capacity they lose."

The message is clear. No matter what your age, expect the worst and that's what you're likely to get. So, why not expect the best—and exercise?

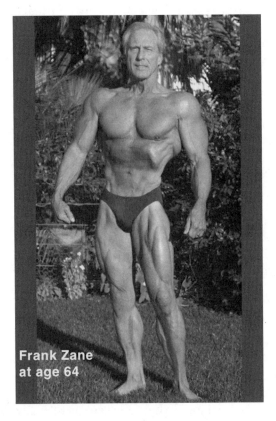

Frank Zane
at age 64

Three-time Mr. Olympia, Frank Zane expects to celebrate all of his birthdays between now and 70 looking better than he does here, at 64. Don't bet against him. *Photo courtesy of Frank Zane*

Exercise and Well-Being

People who feel good about themselves and their life are more likely to be physically active and exercise regularly. And when you exercise, you are more likely to feel a sense of well-being.

It's a win-win deal.

The physical effects of exercise are well known: increased blood flow to the brain, production and regulation of hormones, release of endorphins, and reduction of stress and anxiety. The psychological effects are less well-known, so let's talk a bit about the emotional connection between exercise and well-being.

A feeling of mastery is probably the most obvious emotional effect of exercise. In the words of Dr. Spirduso and her co-authors, "Increases in physical strength, endurance, and ability provide individuals with a feeling that they have more control over their environment and, thus, they are less vulnerable."

There is also a people connection. Many adults get a psychological boost by exercising with friends or in a formal program, perhaps at a community center or a commercial health club. Some program directors say the social contacts may be almost as desirable as the health benefits. The approval and encouragement of group participants or outside family and friends makes people feel better and more in control. The other side of the coin is that some people may prefer to exercise alone and suffer a psychological detriment in a group setting. Spirduso et al. say that the need for social interaction is highly individual.

Lastly, the distraction hypothesis holds that "exercise may be considered a diversion from the stresses of daily life." I offered a somewhat similar view in the Training Psychology section of my book Ripped 2: "It's important to have a sanctuary where we're in control, even if it's only in the gym. The hour or so I spend in the gym calms me for the rest of my day. Controlling the stress that I undergo in my gym fortifies me for the chaos on the outside."

Take it from me: nothing improves your outlook on life like a good workout. When things go well in the gym, the whole world looks better.

Upper Limits of Physical Performance

Many others share my enthusiasm for pushing the envelope in sports and exercise. Spirduso, Francis, and MacRae end their book with an upbeat chapter on the performance levels of elite older athletes. "One of the best ways to determine human physical potential throughout the life span," they observe, "is to study athletic performances of individuals at different ages." No matter what the sport, they emphasize that the records for masters athletes are remarkable—and likely to keep going up.

"The most striking example is that for men aged 60 to 69 years the United States record in the [25-mile] cycling road race is only 14% lower than the U.S. record set by young men," they write. Nevertheless, they say, "It is likely that the observed age decrements in the oldest groups are overestimated. Age records have been improving every year as the popularity of masters' competitions increases and more and more people compete." What's more, they add, "most researchers believe that even the most zealous of elderly competitors usually do not train as intensely as young athletes do." As the numbers increase, so too will the fervor—and the results.

Masters athletes "inspire an upward look...and give hope" for everyone, Dr. Spirduso and her co-authors conclude.

The Competitive Edge

A revolution is taking place in our understanding of the aging process. Most people take it for granted that aging means an inevitable physical decline. For years, authorities have said

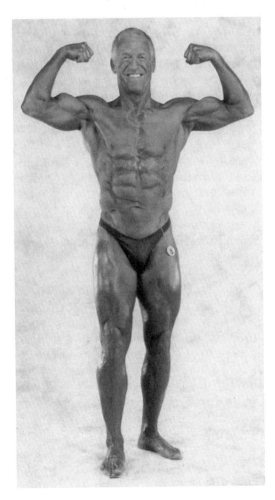

Murrell Hall, 65, shown here, is an example; he ignores stereotypes and has the lean and muscular body to show for it. Weight training since his early 20s, he has competed successfully for 25 years, in more than 100 bodybuilding competitions. *Photo courtesy Murrell Hall*

that after 25 we lose about 1% per year in aerobic capacity, strength, speed, and a whole host of physical attributes. That's just the way it is, gerontologists have maintained. Well, it's now becoming increasingly clear that it doesn't have to be that way. In fact, the 1%-per-year rule of thumb may have little, if any, application to individuals who continue to train at a competitive level.

The late George Sheehan, a cardiologist and my favorite fitness philosopher, wrote about Dr. Michael Pollock's study of 24 healthy, active men (including Sheehan) who continued to train after the normal competitive period.

At the beginning of the study in 1971, all were 40 and high-level athletes, mostly runners. Ten years later, when Pollock tested the men again, he found that those who had continued to train hard showed much less deterioration.

Surprisingly, at least to adherents of the old rule of thumb, the men who continued to train for high-level competition maintained their ability to consume oxygen (an important gauge of fitness); over the 10-year period of the study, their oxygen consumption (VO2 Max) barely declined. Those who allowed training intensity to drop off, however, showed a marked decline over the same period; their VO2 Max declined by an average of 12.5%, compared to a decline of only 1.7% for the competitive group.

With every year that goes by support continues to build for Pollock's finding that the key to holding off the aging process is consistent hard training. For example, my friend Richard Winett, PhD, a professor of health psychology at Virginia Tech and editor of *Master Trainer* newsletter (ageless-athletes.com), called my attention to a highly encouraging study involving tens of thousands of male swimmers, who compete in 5-year age brackets, from 25 to 75.

Here's a summary of the results: For men who swim regularly, physical decline begins not at 25, but in the mid-30s. In fact, these men were actually faster in their early 30s than in their late 20s. Decline began almost imperceptibly for these swimmers. They do not decline at the 1% per-year rate until they reach their early 70s.

"This is a dramatic finding," lead researcher Phil Whitten, PhD, wrote in *Swim* magazine. It means that the 1%-decline-per-year-after-age-25 rule applies only to those who lead a sedentary lifestyle; they lose 25% of their physical capacity by the age of 50 and by 75 they have lost 50%.

In contrast, if you swim regularly—and competitively—the decline is only 3.5% by the age of 50 and 19.1% by age 75. Another way to look at it is a 70-year-old competitive swimmer will have the strength and vitality of a "normal" 45-year-old.

Moreover, Whitten is convinced that his results actually understate what is theoretically possible: "Almost all of the decline, I believe, is due to a sedentary, unhealthy lifestyle." Most masters swimmers have families and job responsibilities, Whitten observed. They are unable to train more than an hour or so a day. "Were they able to put in the time and mileage top collegiate swimmers do, they probably could swim even faster."

Like Pollock (and Spirduso), Whitten believes the secret to maintaining performance with advancing age is to keep training and challenging yourself. He speculates that the comeback attempt by swimmer Mark Spitz, much-publicized at the time, failed not because of age, but because Spitz took a 16-year break from training after his seven-gold-medal performance at the 1972 Olympics. Whitten calculates, based on his study of older swimmers, that a 42-year-old Spitz would have been capable of swimming slightly faster than his world record 20 years earlier—"if he'd never stopped [swimming] at all after Munich."

That's a big *if*, but it suggests what's possible. I've never stopped training and trying to improve. So it can be done.

The ideal is to start early and keep training. But it's never too late. If you stopped, or never started, begin now.

Nothing is accomplished by crying over spilled milk, or worrying about what may happen far into the future. You can't change the past or control the future, but you can do something about the present.

Here's the story of an elite strength athlete who understands the importance of staying in the present.

Focus on Now

With one event to go in the 2006 MET-Rx World's Strongest Man competition, Phil Pfister was asked by Bill Kazmier whether he thought he could win the last event and become the first American to win the title since 1982 (when Kazmier won for the third and last time). Pfister, who had just edged out reigning champion Mariusz Pudzianowski of Poland in the Car Walk (by about 10 seconds) and trailed by only 1/2 point in the overall competition, said he couldn't think about that yet, that he wanted to enjoy his event victory over the three-time winner. "All we have is right now," Pfister said with a broad smile. He went on to move ahead of Pudzianowski on the fifth and last Atlas Stone, and make good on his vow five years earlier to win the premier strongman title "one day."

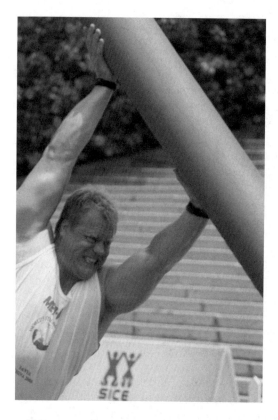

Phil Pfister manhandles a series of progressively heavier Fingers in the 2006 MET-Rx World's Strongest Man competition. *Photo courtesy of IMG Media.*

Pfister, a fireman from West Virginia, has been training his entire adult life to become the World's Strongest Man, and no doubt intends to defend the title as long as he can. He probably has little time or inclination to think about what will happen when he is no longer competitive. Two other amazing athletes have talked about that prospect, however, and expressed much the same thought as Phil Pfister did on the eve of his magnificent victory. Both are endurance athletes who have devoted their lives to pushing their limits.

Dean Karnazes' quest is to run longer and farther than anyone else. His main strength is that he never gives up. You can read about how he goes from one challenge to another, each more outrageous than the last, in his book, *Ultra Marathon Man* (2006, Tarcher/Penguin). His latest ultra challenge—to run 50 marathons in 50 days in 50 states—was featured in the October 2006 issue of *Runner's World.* Author Cynthia Gorney asked him many interesting questions, but the one that caught my attention was how he plans to cope with the time in his life when, because of "age or overreaching or both," he encounters a goal he can't meet. After a long thoughtful pause, he responded: "I can't go there. I'm still so stuck on putting one foot in front of the other that I haven't begun to reflect on what's going to happen when I can't go any farther." He then said something about finding a new adventure, but his bottom line is the same as Pfister's: Focus on the here and now.

Dave McGillivary is a miniature (he stopped growing early, at 5 feet 4 inches) but equally determined version of Dean Karnazes. At 24, he completed a solo run of 3,452 miles across the United States to raise funds for the Jimmy Fund, the official charity of the Boston Red Sox. He now specializes in organizing and managing mass-participation events throughout the US and abroad. His most visible position is race director of the Boston Marathon.

In his inspiring book, *The Last Pick* (2006, Rodale), he tells about his obsession with repetitiveness. (He says it runs in his family.) "The best example," he writes, "is that each year on my birthday, since turning 12, I have run my age in miles. This past year, I ran 51 miles to celebrate my 51st year." He also runs the Boston Marathon every year, even though his race responsibilities now require that he start after the last runner finishes.

"I must admit that, when the day comes—and it will—that either one of these ends, there is going to be a void in my life too big to fathom." Like Pfister and Karnazes, he simply can't afford to dwell on that now. Nevertheless, he's already starting to think about changing the rules on his birthday run. "Maybe I'll start counting backward and begin subtracting miles as I get older, or perhaps I'll use a new formula in which each decade equals 1 mile," he writes. The question remains, nevertheless, what will he do when he can no longer meet the challenge?

He answers that question at the very end of the book: "I will keep going until some higher power decides it's time for me to stop." In short, he'll cross that bridge when he comes to it. "At the end of my life," he continued, "I'd like to think I gave everything I had and then some, right up until I simply run out of time."

Another answer to our question, perhaps the clearest of all, comes from my friend Steve Chandler's book The Story of You (2006, Career Press). Chandler's basic premise is that the stories we tell about ourselves can be the most false and limiting part of our lives. "People's internal stories about themselves are almost always negative because they've been programmed that way," he writes.

In the final chapter he tells about Billy, who had attended one of his seminars "about leaving your victim story behind and owning your life." Billy had a "valid" victim story: he had a brain tumor. Nevertheless, to Chandler's surprise and delight, the seminar made him realize that he had a choice how to respond to his malady.

He stopped being a victim and confronted his doctor with the ineffectiveness of his pain medication. He insisted that the doctor give him something that worked. In a matter of days Billy was on a completely different pain management program, one that worked.

"I'm pain free," he told Chandler, smiling. "At least for today. But that's enough for me! Who has more than today?"

Make every day count. As I said earlier, expect and work for the best, and that's what you'll get—almost all the time.

* * * *

In this chapter, we talked about great expectations, mine and yours. Attitude matters. If you think you can, you will probably succeed. Nothing can be gained from negative thinking. We feel better, look better, and are better when we stay positive, continue to challenge our upper limits, and focus on the here and now.

In spite of our best efforts, however, things don't always work out the way we hope and expect. There will be some bumps in the road. Recently, I've had to deal with two common medical problems; chances are that you will (or have) encounter(ed) similar obstacles at some time in your life. Let's talk about overcoming.

Special note to readers: After reading about the power of great expectations, some of you are probably not in the mood to hear about bumps in the road; you want to move on to more exciting topics. If that's you, move on to Chapter Three, and come back to the next chapter when you're ready. I'll tell you now, however, that the chapter on overcoming is upbeat and ends on a happy note.

"It's not how hard you can hit. It's how many hits you can take and keep moving forward."

Rocky Balboa

Chapter Two

Overcoming

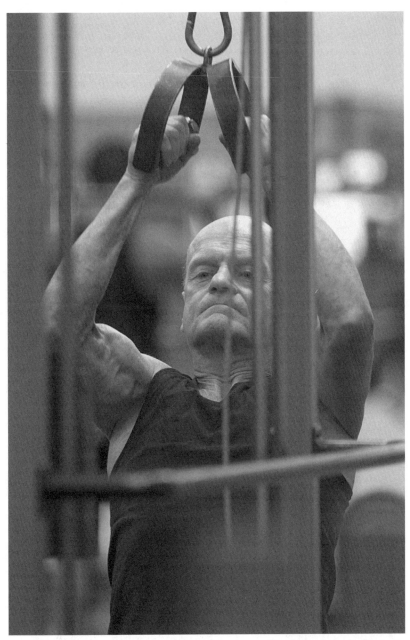

Photo by Laszlo Bencze

Learning and Growing

The next few sections are about some of the high (and low) points of the two surgeries I mentioned earlier, and how I coped with medical adversity for the first time in my life. I made some mistakes along the way, but I learned and grew from both experiences.

The purpose of telling you about these medical problems is to convey three main messages:

- Your fitness level going into a medical problem is likely to have a major impact on the final outcome.

- You don't have to take your care or your situation at face value. Unless you require immediate attention, you are in charge. Speak up for yourself. Ask questions.

- Ultimate responsibility resides with you. It's up to you to do everything possible to help yourself.

You've got a Problem!

My regular health and fitness evaluation at the Cooper Clinic in Dallas revealed that I was retaining an unusual amount of urine. Dr. McFarlin recommended that I have the condition evaluated, so I scheduled an appointment with a well-regarded local urologist.

I'd never been to a urologist and didn't know what to expect. Since Dr. McFarlin had found that my prostate is not enlarged, I didn't see my problem as any big deal. Had I known what was coming, I would've been more concerned.

The urologist, a man of few words, scanned a long questionnaire I had completed prior to the exam, along with McFarlin's report. He asked me a few questions about both.

Without further ado, he did a "vigorous" rectal exam, confirming Dr. McFarlin's finding that my prostate is normal in size. He didn't explain what he was doing (a pattern as it turned out), but I knew from past experience.

The next procedure was new to me, however. Again without explanation, he spread some lubricant on my lower abdomen and passed a wand back and forth several times. What happened next was certainly a surprise.

He read off some numbers that meant nothing to me, and said sternly, "You've got a problem." Startled, I asked what he meant. He explained that the numbers were the volume of urine in my bladder; it was apparently a lot.

Telling me to take a deep breath and relax, he inserted an instrument up through my penis to look inside my bladder—an unanticipated and uncomfortable experience. "See anything unusual?" I asked. "No," he answered, "nothing that would explain the urinary retention."

Before leaving, I stopped the doctor in the hall and asked what he thought might be causing my problem. He said he didn't know but that the urine flow tests, which had been scheduled, might provide some clues. Almost in passing, he added that patients retaining that amount of urine often had to catheterize themselves three or four times a day to control the problem. He didn't offer any further explanation.

A few days later I returned to hear the results of the flow tests. The doctor said the tests confirmed that I was retaining a copious amount of urine, but not much more. He then repeated his previous comment about self-catheterization, adding: "That's my recommendation." (Again, no explanation.) Having had time to consider that solution and the effect it would have on my quality of life, I was ready with my response: "I'm not going to do that, unless it's absolutely necessary." (I thought I'd been coping okay.)

He looked a bit stunned. I don't think he was accustomed to having his recommendations challenged.

Instead of going home with a catheter in hand, the search for the cause of my distended bladder continued.

Kissing Lobes

"Why not just follow the situation along?" I asked. "It doesn't seem to be causing any serious trouble."

"We don't know that," the doctor replied. He explained (finally) that urine backing up in my bladder could damage the kidneys. "You could also end up with a 'floppy bladder' [a loss of tone in your bladder]," he added. "We better get an ultrasound of your kidneys and prostate."

Convinced that the situation might be more serious than I thought, I agreed. "Fine, let's do it."

Two weeks later, I was back for the ultrasound.

"Your kidneys are right where they're supposed to be, and no fat to blur the image," the pleasant and self-assured female technician reported. "They look good, no problems that I can see. Now, let's look at your prostate...It's not enlarged." I said, "That's good." She agreed. But then, the tone of her voice changed, becoming more serious. "You've got lobes on top of your prostate; I see a lot of men with the same thing," she said calmly. "That's something new," I commented. "The doctor will probably want to talk to you about that," she added. "I'll bet he will," I replied.

She showed me the image on the computer screen. It looked

like two mounds sitting side-by-side on top of my prostate, apparently pressing or protruding into my bladder. It was quite a sight. I felt sure we'd found the problem.

A short time later, I was sitting in the examining room, waiting for the doctor. When he appeared, I said: "I guess we've found the problem." He looked at me blankly, and said nothing. Apparently, he had not seen or been told about the ultrasound results. He proceeded to examine the film, moving from frame to frame. I waited for him to see what the tech had shown me earlier. "Whoa," he said when he spotted the abnormal formations. He called them "kissing lobes." He explained that the lobes are in the area where the urine drains from the bladder through the prostate.

"That's the problem, right?" I asked again. "Probably, but we can't be sure," he answered. He took the film to show one of his partners. "We think removing the lobes is worth a try; we can't guarantee it will solve the problem, but we believe it will help."

I called Dr. McFarlin that afternoon and explained what had happened. He was familiar with "kissing lobes" and confirmed everything I had been told (except the self catheterization part, which he agreed was "no way to live"). The technician was correct that kissing lobes are common, but usually on enlarged prostates. My case was a bit unusual, because my prostate is otherwise normal.

McFarlin encouraged me to have the surgery. "You're so healthy otherwise, think of solving this problem as maintenance to make sure you stay that way," he counseled. He said there was no hurry, to have the surgery when it fit my schedule. He added, "Remember that you're in charge."

I called the urologist's office, and the surgery was scheduled.

Shaken Expectations

The last time I had surgery was in the fourth grade when I shot myself in the knee. I dreaded going into the hospital. Hospitals can be dangerous places, with all the ailing people and the prospect of contracting a staph infection. Not to mention hospital food.

I certainly didn't look forward to having a rather large instrument inserted through my penis for the purpose of chopping and burning off the top of my prostate. And those darn catheters. Lance Armstrong wrote in his book that one of the most painful incidents in his long struggle with cancer was having the catheter removed. My Dad also had a bad experience with a catheter in the hospital. Well, those things turned out to be nowhere near as bad as I imagined. Moreover, the food was pretty good. I actually enjoyed it for a few days (along with food Carol brought in for me).

My hospital experience was no picnic, mind you, but certainly not terrible. The worst part was getting my drainage system going again after the catheter was removed. I was motivated, because I *really* didn't want to be sent home with a catheter in place. It was a close call, but I left the hospital sans catheter.

Frankly, I was treated very well. The nurses—all of them—were wonderful. The high point was having a fit-looking nurse recognize me in the recovery room; she'd seen my photos in *Muscle & Fitness*. She commented on how good I looked. Considering the circumstances that was a bit of a stretch, but it made me feel good anyway. I autographed a book for the nurse and her husband. Again, I was treated very well.

The most troubling aspect was having my expectations shaken. As Carol observed, the whole situation went against my experience so far and my optimistic view of the future. I expected a few problems to come with aging, but frankly I didn't expect this so soon. I went to the doctor with what I considered a minor problem—and ended up in surgery.

I was probably the healthiest person in the hospital. One nurse, a kind and caring older lady, asked how long I'd been sick. I snapped back, "I'm not sick." But there I was thrown in with a bunch of *sick* people. It just didn't seem right. Darn it, I didn't belong there, and I wanted out ASAP. I came away feeling more vulnerable than before, my rose colored glasses a little cloudy for the first time.

Fortunately, about that time I received a long hand-written letter from Roy Rose, an old friend from Australia, which helped me regain perspective. As luck would have it, he was relaxing at home recovering from prostate surgery three days before—and feeling good, philosophical, about the whole experience. The surgery had gone well. "No problems at all," he wrote. "Hopefully, now trips to the loo will be less frequent and more productive," he added matter-of-factly. What he said next was exactly what I needed to hear: "Coming during the great run I've had my whole life with excellent health, this is but a mere hiccup."

If anything I should be thanking my lucky stars—and my healthy lifestyle.

Unfortunately, I was not done with catheters. First, however, I want to tell you about my hip problem and eventual surgery.

Twinge in Hip

In the summer and fall of 2004, I began to feel something going on in my right upper thigh, especially when walking downhill.

It would come and go, and I didn't think much about it. And then I came back from a walk one evening in late November to discover that going up the step into our house hurt my hip. It was strange, but still no big deal. I didn't pay much attention to it, because it didn't interfere with my workouts. I could squat and deadlift without pain. It began to bother me more and more, however, especially when going up stairs or lifting my leg to get into a car.

I didn't do anything about it—until March of 2005 when I noticed a clearly-defined swollen area where my groin and upper thigh intersect. It didn't hurt, but it sure got my attention. After a CT-scan showed that the swelling in my groin was most likely caused by drainage from my hip, Dr. Matt Rounseville, my primary care physician, sent me to Robert Wilson, MD, a sports medicine orthopedist.

In a matter of minutes, Dr. Wilson told me I had osteoarthritis of the right hip. After five weeks of conservative treatment failed to cure my hip, we decided together that I needed a hip replacement.

That's when the real adventure began.

Dan Sawyer and the Anterior Approach

Judge Dan Sawyer, a resident of Shreveport, Louisiana, and I have met only once, in 2004, but we've been corresponding since 1992, perhaps longer. Dan has been watching his diet and exercising his whole life and looks much younger than his years. He's a great friend.

Dan told me about the anterior approach to hip replacement. He has had both hips replaced, first the traditional way and about two years later using the anterior approach. After his first hip, Dan says he felt like a mummy and couldn't turn over in bed without help for about eight days. With the new method, he went into the hospital on Thursday morning and was released about noon on Saturday. "With the new approach," Dan told me after learning that I needed a hip replacement, "you'll have so little pain you'll forget to complain."

The basic difference is that the new approach causes less tissue damage, making recovery faster and less painful. The surgeon goes in from the front and through a natural opening; no major muscles are cut. The thigh and hip muscles remain intact. There is almost no chance of dislocation, because the muscles are still working to stabilize the hip joint, just like before the operation. The technical name for the new procedure is "minimally invasive anterior approach."

Joel Matta, MD, who pioneered and perfected the approach in

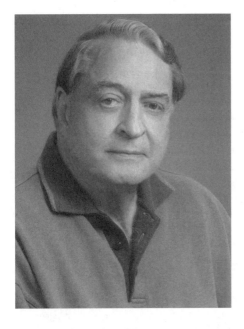

Dan sent us this photo taken in the period between his two hip replacements, the first using the traditional approach and the second the anterior approach. He insists that he looks a lot younger now, after the new procedure.

this country, says a special table is the key to doing an anterior approach. The table is used to rotate, lower, and extend the patient's leg, exposing the hip joint.

I told Dr. Wilson about the new approach. After we determined that no one in New Mexico does the procedure, he encouraged me to look outside the state for a doctor using the method taught by Dr. Matta.

With the help of a list of doctors in adjoining states provided by Dan Sawyer's surgeon (Cambize Shahrdar, MD), I did some research on the Internet and zeroed in on Swiss-born Stefan Kreuzer, MD, who learned the procedure from Dr. Matta and practices in Houston. Kreuzer is second only to Matta in anterior approach surgeries performed.

Doctor Kreuzer

Kreuzer is an extremely busy man. Nevertheless, on our first visit, he walked into the examining room where Carol and I were waiting, calmly sat down and listened to us like we were his one and only concern. "If you took the time to come here to see me, I've got as much time as necessary to discuss your problem," he told us. I decided in a matter of minutes that he was the guy to do my hip. Carol, an astute judge of character, usually takes longer to decide, but she readily agreed.

During that first appointment with Dr. Kreuzer, I emphasized that I expected to continue hard training, weights and aerobics, after having my hip replaced, recognizing, of course, that some adjustments might be necessary. He promised to "make some calls" to determine the best hip to meet my requirements.

Several weeks later, I received a call from Kreuzer. He explained the basic choices and outlined the pros and cons of each option. His favorite, he said, was the Oxinium femoral head. He said it was probably the best option "in view of my exercise habits." He gave me the name of the company that developed the head, UK-based Smith & Nephew, and suggested that I check it out and let him know. I was impressed. That told me he was making a special effort to meet my needs.

Hip replacements with the Oxinium head "could last twice as long as standard devices," says a Smith & Nephew News Release. "Compared to the traditional implant, Oxinium is 4,900 times more resistant to abrasion, 160 times smoother and twice as hard."

There's more to an implant than the head, of course. Hip implants have three components: A socket cup, a femoral head, and a stem that fits into thigh bone, the femur. The socket cup wears faster if the surface of the head is scratched or roughened.

The cup recommended by Kreuzer is made of polyethylene, a form of plastic. The Smith & Nephew News Release says, "Even a single scratch on the surface [of the head] can increase the rate of plastic wear by 10 times, and substantially reduce the life span of an implant." That, of course, makes the wear-resistant properties of the Oxinium head extremely important.

An Oxinium head in a polyethylene socket liner, both made by Smith and Nephew, sounded good to me.

But Kreuzer wasn't done looking for the best combination. He called me in the holding area at the hospital on the morning of the surgery to say he'd found a better socket cup made by Stryker Orthopaedics, a U.S. company, and that it was on the way. He said I'd be well rewarded for waiting a few extra hours for it to arrive. So Carol and I waited.

The surgery, originally scheduled for 8:30 AM, didn't get under way until about 12:30. Seeing patients (and their loved ones) come into the holding area, and then wheeled off to the operating room all morning was like being on the set of *General Hospital*. Kreuzer drew a picture of the new cup (thinner, but stronger, with substantially more surface) on a paper towel for us shortly before I was wheeled off into the operating room. The last thing I remember is getting a glimpse of the special table.

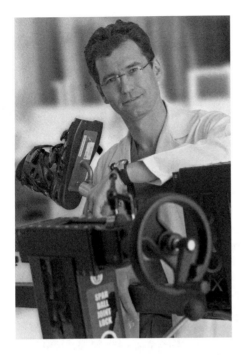

Dr. Stefan Kreuzer and the business end of the special table; you can see the boot for the patient's foot.
Photo courtesy of Stefan Kreuzer

Miracle in Houston

With two relatively minor exceptions (which I will explain shortly), the anterior approach has lived up to Dan Sawyer's promise. The extra effort and expense to find Dr. Kreuzer has been well rewarded. My recovery has been amazing, almost a miracle. I have a sturdy new hip and a new lease on life.

Carol and I flew into Houston Sunday afternoon, and I checked into Memorial Hermann Memorial City Hospital the next morning. I was out of recovery and in my room about 6 that evening. By 9, the nurse had me out of bed and on my feet. I was able to put full weight on my new hip, with no pain. I then made a full lap around the orthopedic wing with the aid of a walker. I was a little uncomfortable and shaky, but had nothing that could be called pain.

The next morning I was walking with a cane, again with some discomfort but no pain. A physical therapist had me do some exercises and showed me how to navigate stairs with a cane. He also gave me "A Patient's Guide to Rehab after Anterior Total Hip Replacement." Later that morning, Dr. Kreuzer came by to see me. After we talked, at my request, he jotted a progressive week-by-week exercise rehab plan on a paper towel. Knowing that I'm more eager than most patients, he added, "I won't be disappointed if you do less."

23

After lunch, Dr. Zoran Cupic, Kreuzer's partner, who assisted in the surgery, came in to check my incision, and asked if I wanted to go home. I did, of course. I was released from the hospital at mid-afternoon—almost exactly 24 hours after completion of the surgery.

This was a little faster than usual, probably due to my physical condition (more on that below), but not much. The typical hospital stay after the new procedure is two to three days, according to the doctors' office.

Carol and I were back in our hotel room by dinner time.

On Wednesday, I practiced walking in the hallway with a cane. The next morning, Carol and I took a walk outside, with me still using the cane. That afternoon I went up and down the stairs in the hotel, again with aid of the cane.

On Friday morning, before my first post-op appointment, I walked without the cane for the first time. At the doctors' office, I absent-mindedly left the cane in the X-ray room! The technician walked down the hall and returned it to me in the examining room, where Carol and I were waiting to see Dr. Cupic. Forgetting the cane was a good sign, they said. We thought so too. (According to Dr. Matta, the median time of first walking without an assistive device is eight days.)

I used a cane to walk through the airports, but needed no other assistance. Carol and I were home in Albuquerque on Friday evening. Our trip to have my hip replaced, round trip, took a few hours over five days.

I used a cane to walk in the street in front of our house on Saturday—but never used the cane again. (The median time when patients *stop* using an assistive devise, according to Matta, is 15 days.) On Sunday, six days after the surgery, I walked down and up the two flights of stairs in our house, *without favoring my new hip or using the handrail.* I did the stairs five times on Monday and 10 the following day.

I was stiff, of course, and sore. It would be next to impossible to extract my old hip and put in a new one without inflicting some trauma. I was working with bruised and stretched muscles, and complete recovery would require more time.

Dr. Kreuzer said "no lower-body weight training for six weeks," to give the bone time to grow solidly around the new joint. Otherwise, I was free to resume normal activities.

I saw Dr. Wilson for my 6-week follow-up exam. "Clarence is doing quite well at this time, progressing through his physical therapy as prescribed and now gradually getting back to training," he wrote in a file note provided to Dr. Kreuzer and Dr. Rounseville.

My only problem was that my hip flexors were not coming back as fast as I expected. Both Kreuzer and Wilson urged me to "take it easy" and give my body time to rebuild the strength and range of motion in this area. As I will explain shortly, my right hip flexors were the only muscles debilitated prior to the surgery.

At 6-months, Wilson wrote: "Clarence, now 68 years of age, is feeling and appearing quite fit having recovered very well from his right total hip replacement. His surgical scar at this point is normal, about three inches long and well-healed. He has developed good strength in the gluteus and hamstrings, the quadriceps, the abductors and adductors of right hip. He walks without a limp and he has a range of motion which is nearly equal that of his normal left hip. ASSESSMENT: Excellent result.

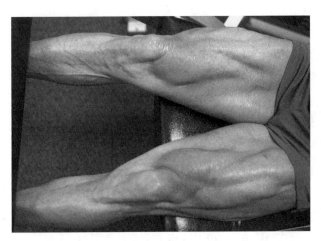

My quads 18 months after hip replacement.
Photo by Laszlo Bencze

My only complaints then—and now—are some numbness in my upper thigh and strength deficit in my hip flexors. My hip works fine; the numbness has no effect on function and the hip flexor problem is minor. I wish these side-effects would go away, of course, but Dr. Kreuzer believes they may be permanent. Dr. Matta says some permanent numbness in the area of the incision is not unusual, but the rest usually goes away with time. I may be an exception.

This is one case where my training apparently worked against me. Dr. Kreuzer says separating and stretching my large muscles apparently caused some nerve damage.

About My Rehab

Frankly, I don't know why my hip went bad. No one can say with certainty. Many factors were probably involved. Fifty-plus years of steady training may have simply taken a toll on my hip. On the other hand, many athletes have their hip or knee replaced decades earlier. For example, 1996 U.S. figure skating champion Rudy Galindo had both hips replaced at age 33. (Galindo is now skating again; he tours with Champions on Ice.) My hip might've gone out earlier without training. Again, no one knows.

My training was clearly a benefit when I needed a hip replacement.

Many patients, perhaps most, come to hip replacement surgery in a debilitated condition. Their muscles are weakened from pain and disuse. Understandably, they avoid movements that hurt. "This leads to an imbalance where the stronger muscles become shorter, thereby stretching and lengthening the weaker muscles," says a handout I received from the rehab people at the hospital. "These imbalances change the way the hip joint usually works. An imbalance of the hip muscles can significantly affect the way you walk or perform other physical activities." This makes rehabilitation take longer. In addition to recovering from the surgery, strength must be rebuilt and imbalances corrected; the patient basically has to learn to walk and move again. I managed to avoid that problem almost entirely.

I avoided movements that hurt before the surgery, but still managed to preserve most of my muscle mass. As noted, it hurt to walk more than a short distance, climb stairs or lift my leg to get in a car—but not to squat. I worked my lower back, hips, and hamstrings using the Glute Ham Developer made by Bigger Faster Stronger in Salt Lake City, Utah (see photo below), and my thighs by squatting and doing leg extensions. The only muscles that suffered were those that pull my right leg and knee forward and up—the hip flexors. The movement that hurt most was lifting my leg to get in the car, especially the high seat in our Jeep. Those muscles were sore and weak, and had to be rehabbed. My lower back, hip, and thigh muscles, however, where many hip-replacement patients have imbalance problems, were in good shape going into the surgery.

As already noted, the only continuing negatives are numbness in my upper thigh and weakness in my hip flexors, probably related to stretching of the large tensor muscle in my upper thigh during the surgery. A less active person probably wouldn't notice the weakness. When I go up stairs two-at-a-time, which requires considerable hip-flexor action, I can't tell the difference between the right hip and the left hip. I am aware of the numbness, but it doesn't affect function. All in all, I've had an excellent result.

I've experienced a minor miracle, thanks to my training and Dr. Kreuzer.

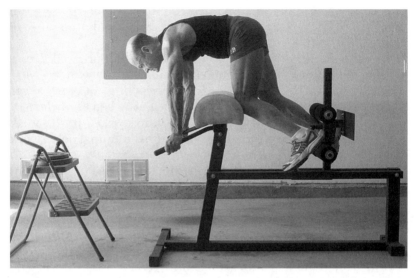

This is the Glute Ham Developer I used before the surgery, and again when I resumed training. We'll discuss its use in Chapter Eight.

Photo by Laszlo Bencze

For many more details on the minimally invasive anterior approach to hip replacement, visit Dr. Matta's website (www.hipandpelvis.com) and Dr. Kreuzer's website (www.anteriorhip.net).

Tale of the Catheter

A little more than a year after the surgery to remove the kissing lobes from my prostate, I again began having trouble emptying by bladder; scar tissue forming at the site of the surgery was apparently restricting the passageway. It was scary; I didn't want to be forced to go to the hospital Emergency Room to get relief. To avoid that, I reluctantly decided to go back to the urologist's office and have them teach me how to catheterize myself—something I had resisted from my very first visit. Unfortunately, things got a lot worse after that—before they got a whole lot better.

Believe me, I wouldn't be telling about this if there wasn't a powerful—and positive—message at the end of the story. Here's what happened.

Milton, a very nice man at the urology office, was assigned to teach me how to do something most males dread. After I tried to insert the catheter, and failed, he tried over, and over—and failed. I ended up in the ER after all, where my doctor's partner spent the better part of an hour trying to catheterize me—and also failed. The passageway was obviously blocked. It makes me cringe to write about it now.

I was again scheduled for surgery, where my original doctor tried to make his way up through my penis into my bladder—and also failed. I left the hospital with a tube coming out of my lower abdomen emptying my bladder into a bag attached to my leg.

It was a nuisance, but it didn't hurt and worked pretty well, especially considering the alternative. I even managed to work out with the arrangement.

About two weeks later, after the trauma from the first attempt had healed, my doctor tried again, using some special instruments. This time he was successful. But there was a problem: What I had managed to avoid after the original surgery a year ago had become a reality. I left the hospital with a catheter in place to keep the outlet open while healing occurred. Like before, a urine collection bag was attached to my leg. I felt like crying when I got home. But I soon adjusted to sleeping—and working out—with the catheter in place. It was a mess, but certainly not the end of the world.

After about two weeks, I was back in the urology office to have the catheter removed—and learn how to catheterize myself. This time it worked like a charm—nothing to it!

In the course of the whole nightmare scenario, the urologist and I reached a rapprochement. I explained that I didn't appreciate him poking me and other unpleasant things without fully explaining what he was going to do—and why. He said he was sorry, and we shook hands. It was as simple as that. I learned from the experience, and I believe he did as well. His skill as a surgeon extricated me from a dire situation. I appreciated what he had done, and I believe he came to appreciate me as an intelligent and involved patient.

That brought us full circle, back to the subject that soured our relationship in the first place: self intermittent catheterization.

He told me I would have to catheterize myself on a regular basis to keep the scar tissue from forming again. He said I might have to do it for the rest of my life. This time I listened—and understood. I didn't want a repeat of what we'd just been through.

He asked me to start out catheterizing myself three times a day, and monitor the results. I did that for a couple of days. As I had feared, it was oppressive. It dominated my day. I didn't like it one damn bit.

This time, however, he said I was going to tell him how often it would be necessary. In other words, he was going to listen to me, just as I was now listening to him. We were going to work together as a team to find the best solution. Now, that was an approach I could live with. I've been listening to my body for a lifetime. I'm good at it.

Over the course of several weeks, I gradually went to twice a day, to every 18 hours…and finally every other day. I was a little worried about telling him I had moved so fast, but it was working fine—and he went with it. We eventually agreed that two or three times a week would be sufficient, as long as my stream stayed strong.

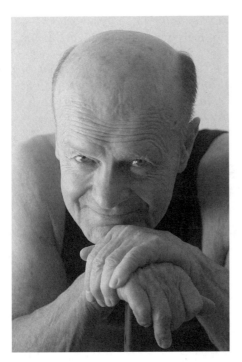

That's quite tolerable, especially to keep me out of the ER or the operating room. It's no big deal—and my urine is flowing like a teenager!

Photo by Laszlo Bencze

* * * *

In this chapter, I told about medical problems I've encountered recently—and overcome. Asking questions and establishing a two-way, cooperative relationship with my urologist helped to resolve the bladder problem. My fitness level played a large part in overcoming my hip problem, both before and after the surgery. Discovering a new approach to hip replacement and locating a skilled and caring surgeon speeded my recovery and return to normal training.

Now, let's turn to a more general topic of interest to just about everyone—losing fat and keeping it off. You've no doubt heard that we're losing the battle and getting fatter all the time. That's true, of course, but it doesn't have to be that way.

"There is probably no biologic reason for men and women to get fatter as they grow older."

Exercise Physiology
McArdle, Katch and Katch (3rd Edition)

In February 1998, when I was 60, on the day of a photo shoot, our Tanita Body Composition Monitor showed my body fat to be 5.5%. As I begin writing this chapter, in my 70th year, my body weight is essentially the same, and my body fat reading is 5.1%.

Chapter Three

Take It Off, Keep It Off

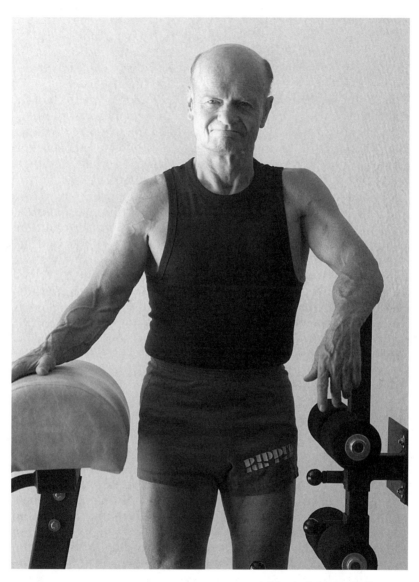

Photo by Laszlo Bencze

The Metabolism Myth

You've heard people say it; maybe you've even said it yourself: "At about 35 my metabolism slowed down, and the fat started to accumulate." The clear inference is that a slowing of metabolism is inevitable, like night follows day. That's simply not true.

Metabolism is the sum of all chemical reactions that take place in the body, including breathing and circulation. Adults do, on average, experience a 2–3% drop in metabolism every ten years, mostly due to a shift in body composition toward fatness.

Body fat deposits also shift. "Not only does percent body fat increase with age, it is slowly and progressively redistributed," says *Physical Dimensions of Aging*, the landmark text cited earlier. "In older adults, intra-abdominal fat tends to increase and subcutaneous fat on limbs tends to decrease." In other words, our bellies grow fatter and our arms and legs skinnier.

The reason, however, is not an aging metabolism.

Exercise Physiology, the excellent text by William D. McArdle, Frank I. Katch, and Victor L. Katch (Lea & Febiger, 3rd Edition, 1991), tells us that people do tend to get fatter with age. College-age men average 15% body fat and older men are usually about 25%. Women in their youth carry body fat of about 25% and move up to 35% or more by age 50. The professors hasten to add, however, that these "average" values should not be accepted as normal. "We believe that one criterion for what is considered 'too fat' should be that established for younger men and women— above 25% for men and above 35% for women. *There is probably no biologic reason for men and women to get fatter as they grow older.*" (Emphasis added)

Increases in body fat, they explain, are more a function of activity than age. Inactivity results in loss of muscle. And loss of muscle, not an aging metabolism, is the primary cause of creeping obesity.

The muscle that remains is as metabolically active as ever. Researchers in the 1940s, led by Dr. Ancel Keys at the University of Minnesota, measured the energy requirements of people of different ages with different amounts of body fat. They found that the energy requirement of fat-free body weight (weight of the body minus the body fat) was remarkably constant for both men and women between the ages of 20 and 60. All the subjects, no matter what their sex or age, burned about 1.28 calories per hour per kilogram (2.2 lbs.) of fat-free body weight, under resting conditions.

McArdle, Katch, and Katch, in the Fourth Edition of their book, published in 1996, reported essentially the same thing: "In comparisons between young and middle-aged endurance-trained men having the same fat-free body mass, measures of BMR [basal metabolic rate] were similar for both groups. In addition, there was an accompanying *increase* in resting metabolism in 50- to 65-year old men who significantly increased their fat-free mass through a program of heavy resistance training. *Such data indicate that regular endurance and resistance exercise can offset the decrease in resting metabolism usually noted with aging."* (Emphasis in original text)

In other words, older people on average burn fewer calories per pound of bodyweight than do younger people. But that's because they are inactive and have less lean body mass.

William Evans, PhD and Irwin H. Rosenberg, MD, confirm this in Biomarkers, their landmark book about controlling the aging process (Simon & Schuster 1991, now available in paperback). If you have a reduced amount of muscle, as most middle-aged people do, your metabolic demand for oxygen and your caloric needs decline. That's because muscle tissue is active tissue requiring nourishment, they explain. Fat is passive, serving mainly as a storage form of body energy. "We feel that older people's reduced muscle mass is almost wholly responsible for the gradual reduction in their basal metabolic rate." (Emphasis added)

Evans & Rosenberg say that this reduction in muscle mass—and the slowing of metabolism that it causes—sets up a vicious cycle. As our muscle mass falls, our calorie needs fall with it. The problem, of course, is that we continue eating the same. "Too many calories coupled with too little exertion, a reduced musculature, and a declining metabolic rate adds up to more and more fat." This cycle, they conclude, will only worsen over time—unless broken by a program that increases muscle and restores lost metabolism.

Diet, of course, helps to control creeping obesity, but it's usually not enough. The main solution for an "aging metabolism" is exercise. Exercise builds muscle, increasing resting metabolism, but it also burns more calories while you exercise, and after exercise you continue to use more calories than at rest. Even mild exercise leaves you burning extra calories an hour later. If you exercise harder and longer, after 12 hours your energy requirements may still be elevated.

McArdle, Katch, and Katch confirm this in their Fourth Edition: "An 8-week aerobic training program for older individuals resulted in a 10% increase in resting metabolism *even though fat-free body mass did not change.* (Emphasis added) This suggests that regular exercise affects factors other than body composition that have a stimulating effect on resting metabolism."

A study by researchers at the University of Colorado at Boulder shed more light on this phenomenon. They found that a reduction in physical activity by ten "habitually exercising" older adults (male and female, ages 62 to 67) caused a substantial drop in resting metabolism—in 5 days. Lead author Christopher Bell, PhD, says the drop may be related to changes in the sympathetic nervous system with age. Aerobic exercise, however, seems to protect against such changes that may negatively impact metabolism. (*Journal of Clinical Endocrinology & Metabolism*, Vol. 89, No. 7, 2004.)

So once you start exercising, don't stop. And don't neglect strength training.

Spirduso and her co-authors say, "Aerobic exercise [is] not an effective intervention for increasing muscle mass because [it] does not provide a strong enough stimulus." Resistance exercise does a far better job of building muscle—and metabolism.

And don't let anyone tell you that you can't increase your muscle size and strength as you get older. Evans and Rosenberg and their colleagues at the U.S. Department of Agriculture's Human Nutrition Center on Aging at Tufts University have found that "the muscles of elderly people are just as responsive to weight training as those of younger people." Startlingly, an 8-week program of strength training by 87- to 96-year-old women confined to a nursing home resulted in a tripling of strength and a muscle-size increase of ten percent.

Their important conclusion: "Much of the loss of muscle as we age is preventable—and even reversible."

It comes down to this: Your metabolism won't slow down if you don't.

Now, let's talk about controlling metabolism—and body weight—with diet. The solution is closer than you may think.

Mother Nature's Amazing Balancing Act

It seems that ads for new weight loss programs appear almost daily. Obviously, the demand is growing. Americans desperately seek a cure for fatness.

In fact, we don't need to wait another day. Our bodies, with a few rare exceptions, already have a marvelous ability to balance calorie intake and expenditure. All we have to do is start working with—rather than against—our biology. It takes a little longer, but the payoff for most people is permanent leanness.

Few of us get fat fast. We get fat very slowly. According to *Physiology of Sport and Exercise*, the beautifully designed textbook by Jack H. Wilmore and David L. Costill (Human Kinetics, Third Edition, 2004), the average person in this country gains one pound each year after age 25, or a total of 30 pounds of excess weight by age 55. But that's not the whole story. We also lose half a pound of fat-free mass (bone and muscle) each year because of reduced physical activity. "Taking this into account, an average person's body fat actually increases by 1.5 pounds each year, or a 45-pound fat gain over a 30-year period!" write Wilmore and Costill.

Sounds unrelenting, I know, like a slow-moving freight train, but considered one day at a time, it's actually quite manageable.

The average gain of 1.5 pounds of fat represents an excess of only 5,250 calories per year (one pound of fat contains 3,500 calories). That's less than 15 calories a day or, as Wilmore and Costill observe, the amount found in one potato chip. Amazingly, even the average sedentary person comes within one potato chip each day of energy balance.

The body's ability to balance energy intake and expenditure to such a remarkable degree has led scientists to propose that bodyweight is regulated around a given set point, similar to the way in which body temperature is regulated. Excellent evidence for this is found in both animal and human research literature, according to Wilmore and Costill.

When animals are force-fed or starved their weights go up or down, respectively. But when they go back to normal eating, they always return to their original weight. The same thing happens in humans.

In an example given by Wilmore and Costill, overfeeding Vermont prisoners resulted in weight gains of 15% to 25%, but their weights returned to original levels shortly after the experiment ended.

Wilmore and Costill explain that the body adapts to major changes in calorie intake by altering metabolism in three areas:

- Resting metabolic rate (60% to 75% of energy expenditure)

- Digestion, absorption, transport and storage of food (about 10%)

- Activity (15% to 30%)

When we go on a very low calorie diet, our metabolism slows down to conserve energy. Conversely, when we overeat our metabolism speeds up to "waste" the surplus calories.

The increased prevalence of overweight and obesity, of course, suggests that the set point can change. Wilmore and Costill say this appears to happen when rats are put on a high-fat diet for over six months. "It is quite possible that an increase in the fat content of the diet and a decrease in physical activity levels allow set-point weight to increase," they conclude.

It seems likely that consistently cutting back slightly on calories and increasing activity levels will restore the original set point.

The body's ability to defend its weight is truly amazing. Food availability and consumption trends suggest that we are eating substantially more calories than a static analysis of our average weight gain would indicate. "Americans are eating more meals outside the home, relying more heavily on convenience foods, and consuming larger food portions," Wilmore and Costill observe. Needless to say, we are also less active.

Imagine: Even in this age of fast food and automation, our body's natural balancing mechanism brings us within a hair's breath of weight equilibrium. If we just help the system a little each day we can achieve absolute balance, and by tweaking it a little more we can create a negative balance—and lose fat.

Let's look at some ways to do that, which are largely common sense, but not common knowledge—and certainly not common practice.

Lose Slowly

As noted, our metabolism slows in response to severe calorie restriction. Robert Robergs, PhD, who did his doctoral work in exercise physiology under Dr. Costill at Ball State University and is now director of the Center for Exercise at the University of New Mexico, says the metabolism slowdown can be as much as 500 calories per day after six weeks on a very low calorie diet. "That's a huge problem," he emphasizes. "It makes it harder and harder for people to lose weight."

That's why my friend Arno L. Jensen, MD, my former doctor at the Cooper Clinic and the person to whom this book is dedicated, urges his patients to lose slowly, not more than half to one pound a week. To convince them Arnie uses a model of five pounds of fat. "That shocks them," he says, because they don't realize how much flesh five pounds of fat represents. He shows them the model and then explains: "You can lose five of these in a year's time by losing [only] a half pound a week. That just really motivates them" to lose slowly. "That makes them feel good," Jensen adds, because people dread severe dieting.

It is common knowledge, of course, that rapid weight losses are usually temporary. A slowed metabolism is one reason why the weight is soon regained. Another reason, according to Wilmore and Costill, is that rapid losses are often mostly water. The body has built-in safety mechanisms to prevent an imbalance in body fluids, so the lost water is eventually replaced.

Similarly, it's not a good idea to limit the quantity of food you eat. Forcing yourself to stop eating before you're full and satisfied doesn't work very well. My observation is that few people can do it for long, and it's not necessary anyway.

As explained in my earlier books, eating a balanced diet of mostly whole foods will usually put your weight on a downward path. You don't have to worry about restricting the amount you eat, because you become full before exceeding your calorie needs. Your body's appetite control mechanism tells you when you've had enough. Dr. Jensen cautions, however, that you must focus on the whole diet, and not just low fat. "America is getting fat eating a low fat diet," he maintains. "People are keen on eating a low fat diet, but forget that low fat diets have calories."

(As I will explain later in this chapter, there is some evidence that eating a moderate amount of "good" fat aids loss of body fat. It's also good for you.)

Exercise Makes It Work

As explained earlier, exercise burns calories and speeds up the metabolism. It also has an appetite curbing effect. Exercise facilitates the body's natural regulatory ability. This was first demonstrated in 1954 by world-renowned nutritionist Jean Mayer. He reported that animals exercising for periods of 20 minutes to one hour per day ate less than non-exercising animals. He concluded from this and other studies that when your activity falls below a certain minimum level, appetite and food intake does not drop a like amount—and fat begins to accumulate. Apparently, this is one reason why the average person gains fat every year. If you're living a sedentary lifestyle it throws the body's appetite control mechanism off, causing you to eat more calories than you expend.

That's not to suggest that lumberjacks, marathoners, cyclists, and other very active people eat less than sedentary individuals. They eat more, of course. The difference is that people who exercise have an easier time balancing calorie intake and energy expenditure. They can eat more without getting fat. Dr. Robergs notes, for example, that Tour de France cyclists maintain or lose weight consuming more than 5000 calories a day.

Now, let's look at an activity that doesn't live up to its billing: slow-pace exercise. Many fitness gurus, past and present, recommend slow, low-intensity exercise for fat burning, giving people the idea that they should confine exercise to a certain range.

Fat Burn Fallacy

According to Wilmore and Costill, low-intensity aerobic exercise does not necessarily burn more fat than high-intensity aerobic exercise. It's true that the body uses a higher proportion of fat

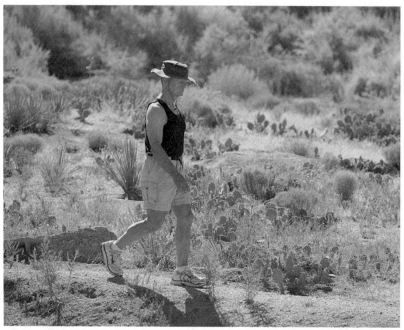

Make walking a regular part of your life and you'll find it easier to control your weight. Do it in pleasant surroundings and enjoy yourself.

Photo by Laszlo Bencze

for energy at lower exercise intensities. However, total calories expended are greater during high-intensity aerobics—and fat burning continues.

For example, an average 40-year-old male will burn the same number of calories from fat exercising for 30 minutes at 50 percent of capacity and at 75 percent. He burns about 145 calories of fat in both cases. Importantly, however, during the higher intensity workout he expends approximately 50 percent more total calories, about 435 compared to only 290 in the course of the low-intensity session.

Dr. Robergs isn't sure how the fat burn fallacy got started, but he believes that people simply like the word "easy." He thinks they grab on to the idea, because it makes training "more readily acceptable." Nevertheless, he says, "you can't convert a relative contribution to an absolute value; it's the total amount of calories [burned] that's most important."

"There is another issue too," Robergs adds, which makes the intensity of the workout all the more important for fat loss. A more intense approach, he explains, "is more conducive to improving the muscle's ability to use fat." The more fit you become, the more likely you are to use fat as fuel.

"When you become more fit," Robergs stresses, "you are just better able to metabolize fat for any given activity you do."

(Some readers, I'm sure, still want to know the intensity level where fat burn level is highest; heck with total calories burned. Here it is, courtesy of Wilmore and Costill: "The fat zone, defined as fat oxidation within 10% of the peak rate, was found to vary from between 55% and 72% of VO2max.")

We've explained why extreme calorie reduction is counterproductive. So, what is the best approach to eating for permanent weight loss? Read on.

How the Masters Eat

The real winners in the battle of the bulge are those who keep the fat off. Anne M. Fletcher, MS, a registered dietitian and former executive editor of *Tufts University Diet & Nutrition Letter*, has made a study of these "masters" of weight control. She located 208 people who lost at least 20 pounds and kept it off for at least three years. Fletcher wrote about her findings in a wonderful series of *Thin For Life* books, which are now available in paperback.

The average weight loss for Fletcher's masters is 64 pounds. The average length of time they have kept off 20-plus pounds is more than 10 years. Fletcher says 30 of her masters have kept off 100 pounds or more!

As you might expect, these people kept the weight off in many different ways. While there is no one right way to lose weight permanently, Fletcher identified five "food secrets of the masters." I have used these techniques for many years (before reading Fletcher's excellent books) and continue to use them to cope with calories. They work.

SECRET #1

Want to be thin more than you want to eat the "wrong" foods. People who stay slim have usually experienced an attitude shift. Fletcher says it's as if a switch flips in their head. They come to a point in life, for one reason or another, where it becomes clear that the benefits of keeping the weight off exceed the costs. As one master told Anne Fletcher, "Nothing tastes as good as being thin feels."

The best example of a profound shift in attitude I've encountered is a 40-year-old, out-of-shape, overweight dentist who called us in 1989 to arrange a consultation after holding his 5-day-old adopted son for the first time. "I knew I had to make some major changes in my life or I wouldn't be around to see him grow up into an adult," he told me.

He now has two adopted boys, both well into their teens. He has stayed in touch with us by phone over the years, and plans to visit for the third time later this year. His weight has fluctuated some, but he has not lost the "spark" for fitness. He's never stopped working to keep his weight down.

When you are truly ready, it's time to move on to the other four food secrets. As you'll see, a firm resolve to keep the pounds off does not imply a lifetime commitment to hunger and deprivation.

SECRET #2

Eat large. The masters focus on the kind of food they eat. Fletcher says most of them eat "by concept" rather than "by number." Only three percent of the masters count grams of fat or calories. What they have learned is how to get the most out of their calories. "They seek out foods that will fill them up but are not fattening," Fletcher explains. In short, they eat large.

The masters have done the homework necessary to learn which foods are high in fat and calories and which are not. They know what to eat and what to avoid. One master told Fletcher he goes by two guiding principles: "First, all foods must be low-fat. (Some fat is good for you and adds satiety.) Second, I eat lots of vegetables and fruits." (Most masters also eat plenty of whole grains and only a little meat, Fletcher says.) Importantly, this master added, "The simple pleasure of eating natural food in its basic form is great."

Calorie for calorie, foods low in fat and high in fiber and water (vegetables, fruits, and grains) are more filling. Why? Because low-fat, high-fiber foods take up more room in your stomach and take longer to eat.

SECRET #3

Fix your full button. My Dad used to say he never let being full stop him from eating. I'm the same way. Many masters are the same way. Eating large solves the problem to a degree, but Fletcher found that the vast majority of her masters "take important steps to place limits on the amount of food they eat."

Masters are careful about portion size. Most of them have learned from long experience to gauge portion size by eye. But if their weight starts creeping up they go back to weighing and measuring portions, especially foods which are higher in calories, such as meat or full-fat dairy products. When I'm being photographed, as I am during the course of writing this book, I measure more things and tighten up on portion sizes. (Details in Chapter 8)

Masters plan their meals. Fletcher says many of them plan meals up to a week in advance. But most importantly, "before they start eating, they decide how much they will serve themselves."

I began using this simple technique about 30 years ago. It has saved me from eating many thousands of excess calories. As related in my earlier books, the only food I put on the table is the food I intend to eat. This keeps in check my inclination to eat everything in sight; I rarely want more than I serve myself initially. (See photos below)

Masters eat consistently. Many told Fletcher they "go out of their way to eat regular meals and avoid skipping meals." Personally, I never miss a meal. That way I don't come to any meal ravenously hungry and out of control; I stay on plan and almost never eat haphazardly.

SECRET #4

If you want it, have it. Most masters "never say never" to fattening foods. In place of hard—and sure to be broken—rules, Ann Fletcher says, "They have control systems for tempting foods so they don't go overboard." They have an escape valve, so to speak, to prevent the buildup of cravings that can easily get out of hand. "Because I don't have any forbidden foods

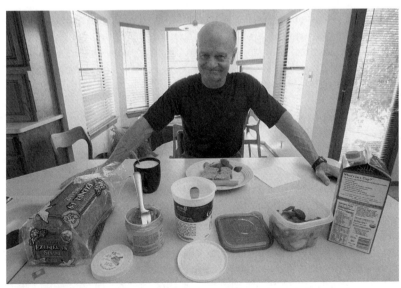

Extra food on the table provides unnecessary temptation and encourages overeating. *Photo by Laszlo Bencze*

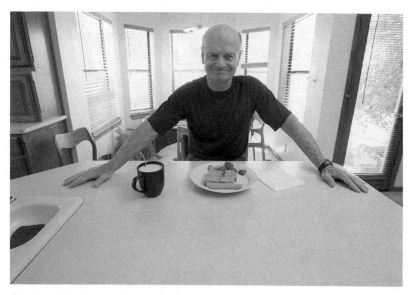

A better idea is to put on the table only what you plan to eat. If you want more, get up and get it—but stop and think about it first. I usually decide I've had all I *really* want. Give it a try and see for yourself.

Photo by Laszlo Bencze

any longer," one master told Fletcher, "I really don't have any problem foods."

I have always urged an *occasional* splurge. When our son Matt was a youngster, one of our favorite father-son activities was going to the ice cream shop. (We didn't go every weekend.) I'd have the biggest, gooiest sundae on the menu and enjoy every bite. But we didn't keep ice cream around the house, and we rarely ate dessert.

Matt, of course, had an occasional cookie or other sweet treat. He's now 34—and lean.

SECRET #5

Don't let the tough times get you down. Everyone's weight control efforts get sidetracked from time to time. For example, you may have problems on vacation or at social events, or at major turning points such as pregnancy, divorce or the death of a loved one, or after quitting smoking. Perhaps you've tried to lose weight repeatedly—and failed time after time. Fletcher's masters have encountered the same problems. In fact, nearly 60 percent tried to lose weight a least five times before they successfully took it off and kept it off.

The masters didn't give up. They used "past" failures as learning experiences, stepping stones if you will, on the way to successful weight control. They picked themselves up and started all over again—each time better equipped to manage the next bump on the road to permanent leanness.

As the masters come to understand, often by trial and error, long-term success comes from eating in a way that registers on your fat cells but not on your mind. That's the subject of the next section.

Mindless Eating

"The best diet is the one you don't know you're on," food psychologist Brian Wansink writes in his insightful book *Mindless Eating* (Bantam, October 2006). "Most people gain (or lose) weight so gradually that they can't really figure out how it happened.

Wansink calls this the *mindless margin*. "It's the margin or zone in which we can either slightly overeat or slightly undereat without being aware of it." This is where most of us gain weight and—ideally—where we can lose weight easily and permanently.

"If we eat way too little, we know it. If we eat way too much we know it," he observes. That's true, isn't it? "But there is a calorie range—a mindless margin—where we feel fine and are unaware of small differences." It's roughly 100 calories over or under calorie equilibrium. Doesn't sound like much, but Wansink says, "Over the course of a year, this mindless margin would either cause us to lose ten pounds or to gain ten pounds."

If we eat 1,000 calories less we feel deprived, and if we eat 1,000 calories more we feel stuffed. Both are uncomfortable—and as a practical matter unsustainable. But 100-200 calories more or less goes unnoticed—and for most people it's the difference between weight gain or weight loss.

Professor Wansink and his graduate students have illustrated mindless eating using something to which we can all relate: movie popcorn. They gave every person who bought a ticket to a movie theater a free soft drink and either a medium-size bucket of popcorn or a large-size, "bigger-than-your-head" bucket. All they asked in return was that the movie patrons answer a few questions.

Both buckets were actually too big for anyone to finish all the popcorn. Plus, because of the time of day, many of the theater patrons had just eaten lunch. The popcorn was also stale. Writes Wansink, "It was stale enough one movie-goer said it was like eating Styrofoam peanuts." That didn't stop anyone from eating it, of course. "During the movie, people would eat a couple of bites, put the bucket down, pick it up again a few minutes later, and continue. It might not have been good enough to eat all at once, but they couldn't leave it alone." (Sound familiar?)

As each person's leftover popcorn was being collected after the movie, they were told: "Some people tonight were given medium-size buckets of popcorn, and others, like yourself, were given these large-size buckets. We have found that the average person who is given a large-size container eats more than if they are given a medium-size container. Do you think you ate more because you had the larger size?"

"Most disagreed." Many added smug comments, such as, "Things like that don't trick me," or "I'm pretty good at knowing when I'm full."

As you probably guessed, what they believed is not what happened.

"Weighing the buckets told us that the big-bucket group ate an average of 173 more calories of popcorn," Wansink reports. "People who were given big buckets ate an average of 53 percent more than those given medium-size buckets. Give them a lot, and they eat a lot."

Wansink and his colleagues have repeated the popcorn study many times—always with the same result. Most people eat mindlessly, based on the size of the container and other cues—not the taste or how hungry or full they are. Within limits, most people don't pay attention to how much they eat.

"Does this mean we can avoid mindless eating simply by replacing large bowls with smaller bowls?" Wansink asks. Yes, that can certainly help. Let me tell you how that worked for me—before I started reading the professor's book.

I'd begun thinking about having photos taken over the course of my 70th year. My weight was stable, but I needed to take off a few pounds to be photo ready. I've done this many times. I never rush the process. I monitor my weight and body fat weekly on my Tanita Body Composition Scale and cut back slightly on my food intake as I zero in on peak condition. I eat regular meals and never let myself get hungry. As indicated above, I want my fat cells to notice but not my mind. One of the adjustments I made involved popcorn.

When Carol and I go to a movie (we go regularly), I usually have a small diet drink and small popcorn, without butter. (Frankly, I don't remember ever buying a large bucket of popcorn; I never ask for butter.) I also have a Tiger's Milk energy bar with the popcorn; Carol and I jokingly call it my candy bar. (It really is good with popcorn.) I have a few kernels of popcorn and a small bite of Tiger's Milk. It's a tasty combination—and has a fraction of the calories of buttered popcorn and a regular candy bar. I've never figured out the calorie difference, but it's a bunch. More importantly, I enjoy every bite and feel quite satisfied, not at all deprived.

Carol noticed that I often leave some of the popcorn. Knowing that I was getting ready for photos, she suggested that I try a junior-size popcorn. After resisting for a few weeks—it's such a dinky looking little container—I gave in and asked for a junior popcorn. Happily, I found that it satisfied me just fine. I didn't know at the time that I was taking a leaf out of Professor Wansink's book, but I can tell you that it works. The small calorie reduction (I haven't calculated the exact number) made no difference in my eating satisfaction. I've been eating the junior popcorn ever since, even after the photos.

That change, along with some other small adjustments in my daily diet and a slight increase in my activity level, started to register in the mirror and my weekly weighings almost immediately. (I'll give some examples of my daily eating pattern in Chapter Seven.)

Now, let's move on to some new ideas about dietary fat and fat loss.

Fat is fattening, but there is some evidence that eating a moderate amount of "good" fat aids loss of body fat. I noted this

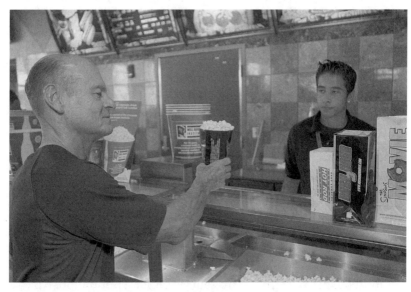

I'm buying my junior popcorn. The theater owners are smart. The bargain sizes shown here on the counter are temptations patrons find hard to resist. *Photo by Laszlo Bencze*

surprising phenomenon in *Challenge Yourself*, but intriguing new details have recently emerged.

"Good" Fat and Fat Loss

The kind of fat you eat seems to be critical.

In a study reported in the December 1996 issue of the journal *Metabolism*, Japanese researchers raised mice prone to diabetes and obesity on a variety of diets containing 60% fat, and then measured the change in body weight. All of the diets contained the same number of calories; the only difference was the type of fat consumed. The resulting variation in weight gain was truly startling.

The difference in weight between the mice fed soybean oil and those fed fish oil was "comparable to the difference in weight between a 225- and a 150-pound man," according to Artemis P. Simopoulos, MD, author of *The Omega Plan* (Harper Collins, 1998). A lard/fish oil comparison produced a weight gain disparity almost as great.

Simopoulos, a highly-regarded authority on fats, noted that soybean oil and lard are high in omega-6 fats and that fish oil is high in omega-3s, but offered no further explanation for the huge difference in weight gain.

Susan Allport provides a detailed and plausible explanation in her book *The Queen Of Fats* (University of California Press, 2006). It's a bit technical, however. Here is my *CliffsNotes™* version. The basic idea isn't hard to grasp.

"There are profound differences between diets and tissues full of omega-6s and omega-3s, differences that slow our bodies down and speed them up," Allport writes.

Analyzing the tissues of animals with different metabolic rates, researchers found that "the fats of large, slow mammals were more saturated and contained more omega-6 fatty acids than the fats of small, fast mammals like the mouse, which contains more DHA," Allport writes. "The fats of high-speed animals like the hummingbird were loaded with DHA." DHA is docosahexaenoic acid, a member of the omega-3 family; it's found in fish.

The high amounts of DHA result in leakier cell membranes— membranes that have to work harder to maintain their integrity. "They have found it is the DHA concentration of membranes that correlates most closely with an animal's metabolic rate," Allport adds.

Metabolism is controlled by genetic factors, but diet also plays a part, which includes the amount of omega-6s and omega-3s an animal eats.

Allport tells us that obesity expert Leonard Storlien, PhD,

was perhaps the first person to see the connection between the "leaky membrane theory" and problems associated with energy balance and obesity. "If you have a person running at a metabolic rate that is 40 percent of someone else," Storlien told Allport in a phone interview, "you would have a profound predisposition for obesity."

"Storlien had already found that rats do develop insulin resistance on diets that were rich in either saturated fats or omega-6s," Allport writes. "But fish oil was different. It protected against both insulin resistance and obesity." This was true in rats, but what about humans?

Storlien knew that the fish-eating Eskimos, studied in the 1970s, had a very low rate of diabetes, and when he heard about the pacemaker or leaky membrane theory immediately saw the "implications for understanding the cluster of diseases surrounding energy and insulin resistance in humans."

Storlien and a group of other researchers looked to the Pima Indians of Arizona, who have the highest incidence of type-2 diabetes in the world, for another human example. They "found half the amount of DHA in the phospholipids of their skeletal muscles as in a group of Australian, largely Caucasian, men," Allport writes. "Skeletal muscle is the major site of glucose uptake in the body, and this difference in DHA content was closely correlated with the Indian's insulin resistance."

Insulin resistance causes the Pimas to store fat—glucose that isn't burned by their muscles is deposited as fat—which is a good thing when food is scarce and unpredictable, but detrimental when food is abundant. "This is a transition that the Pima Indians have recently made," Allport observes. Widespread obesity, regrettably, comes with their newfound abundance.

Unfortunately, neither Storlien nor anyone else has been able to demonstrate improvement in insulin sensitivity among type-2 diabetics after omega-3 fatty acids in their diets are increased. "It's driven most of us nuts," Storlien told Allport. "It happens so easily in animals. Why doesn't it happen in humans?"

The probable reason is that obese people carry huge fat reserves. "It would take years to turn over all of the fats on an obese person [from omega-6 to 3]," Storlien told Allport. "I haven't been able to run my studies out that far. You don't get grants to do long-term intervention studies."

Interestingly, he's had difficulty publishing a one-year study in which a high omega-3 diet did produce "an impressive improvement in insulin action" and other variables. "This study was rejected by five journals," Storlien told Allport. "Not because of the science, but because the reviewers said, 'You couldn't possibly get theses effects from just changing the fatty acid profile of the diet.'"

Metabolism is not a simple matter, Storlien understands. He acknowledges that activity level and calorie intake and many other factors contribute to diabetes and obesity. "But the pacemaker theory is a matter of a number of mechanisms coming together to push metabolism in a particular direction," he told Allport, "and it's time to test it with well-funded, long-term studies."

In the meantime, Allport, Simopoulos, and Storlien say—Eat Fish. Allport also recommends eating lots of fruits and vegetables. Green vegetables, she says, are "full of alpha linolenic acid, the parent omega-3 fatty acid."

As you'll see, that's what I'm doing. Perhaps you should consider doing the same.

Eating fish is probably a good bet, because it's also good for your heart. A Harvard study, published in the *Journal of the American Medical Association* on October 18, 2006, found that people who eat one or two servings of fish per week, especially fatty varieties such as wild salmon, have fewer heart attacks and live longer. (We'll discuss the heart connection in Chapter Six.)

* * * *

In this chapter, I said that lifetime leanness is achievable for the vast majority of people—and explained how and why. Just because most people get fatter as they age doesn't mean it has to be that way. It requires a willingness to help yourself, but staying lean is not as hard as we are led to believe. Taken one day at a time, most people can manage to do it quite well. Be optimistic about becoming lean and staying lean—because you can do it.

In Chapters 5 and 6, I will tell you about the diet and training philosophy that has worked so well for me. Before I do that, however, I want to give you some exciting new information about the health benefits of regular exercise and weight control. Diet and exercise keep you slim and trim and looking good. But the benefits don't stop there. Fitness and leanness have a powerful effect on the length—and especially the quality—of your life.

Let's talk about it next, in Chapter Four.

"Most of what we call aging is decay, and decay is optional; it's under our control.

Henry S. Lodge, MD, co-author
Younger Next Year

"A nearly linear reduction in mortality was observed as fitness levels increased, and each increase of 1 MET in exercise capacity conferred a 12 percent improvement in survival."

Gary J. Balady, M.D.
New England Journal of Medicine

"It is exercise alone that supports the spirit, and keeps the mind in vigor."

Cicero ~65 BC

Chapter Four

Exercise for Life

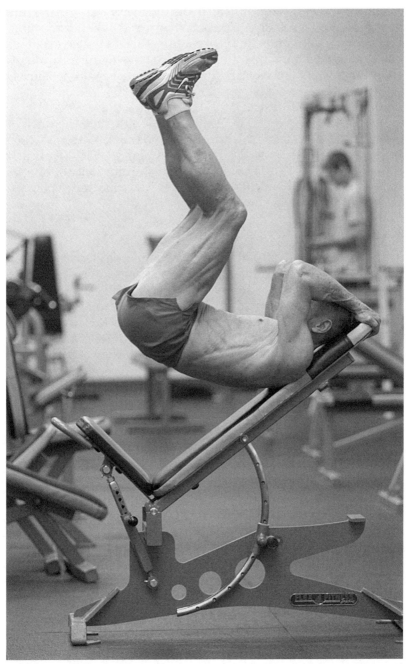

Clarence at Liberty Gym, Albuquerque, NM. *Photo by Laszlo Bencze*

It's in Our Genes

The formula for vibrant health and longevity was written into our genes thousands of years ago. What worked then works now. Life is vastly different now, of course, and that's a problem; but it's one that can be managed. In reality, we have many advantages that our ancient ancestors didn't have. Our comprehension is greater now and we have far more power to control our lifestyle and, therefore, our destiny.

In the next few sections, we'll be talking about the ancient blueprint. It's consistent with my own training pattern, which is explained in Chapters Eight. I didn't plan it that way; it just made sense to me. The ancient mandate is quite logical when we understand the underlying principle. It was a matter of survival then, and that's true now as well.

Exercise Six Days a Week

That's the formula in a nutshell: exercise six days a week. (Stick with me here; this is very important, and very interesting—and less onerous than it sounds.)

A new book does a wonderful job explaining the rationale for the formula and how it can help you survive and thrive in modern times. The book is *Younger Next Year: A Guide to Living Like 50 Until You're 80 and Beyond* by Chris Crowley and Henry S. Lodge, MD (Random House, 2004).

Dr. Henry S. Lodge (Harry) is a board-certified internist who heads a 23-doctor practice in Manhattan. Chris Crowley is a retired lawyer, who was 70 (my age) when the book was published in 2004.

Being a lawyer myself, I like the fact that the book was Chris's idea; Harry was the eager doctor. (How that happened is a good story told in the book.)

Younger Next Year is wide-ranging—it may be the best self-help book ever written on aging well—but I want to focus on a compelling hypothesis Dr. Lodge pulled together from many sources. It provides a firm foundation for the ancient mandate to exercise. The hypothesis is "grow or decay."

Grow or Decay: It's a Choice

Conventional wisdom holds that we begin a long slide into old age and death at about 50. It doesn't have to be that way. You can get off the slippery slope by following the ancient mandate on exercise. How you age is mostly up to you. That's Harry Lodge's premise—and mine.

Harry says changing your lifestyle can eliminate over 50 percent of all illness and injuries in the last third of your life. Furthermore, he says 70 percent of premature death is lifestyle-related. "Even more important," Chris writes in the opening chapter, "is that the *normal* decay associated with aging—the weakness, the sore joints, the lousy balance, the feeling crappy—70 percent of that horror can be forestalled almost until the end."

The "catch," says Harry, is that our body and brain were not designed for modern times. "They were designed for life in nature, where only the fittest survived." That's not new, but Harry adds an intriguing new twist.

"Nature balances growth with decay by setting your body up with an innate tendency toward decay." The signal is weak at first and grows a little stronger each year. Chris calls it the "relentless tide." Between 45 and 55 our bodies switch into a "default to decay" mode. "The free ride of youth is over." Nature's purpose is simple, and brutal: to provide for the next generation. Food was in short supply and needed for the childrearing and productive members of the group.

"In the absence of signals to grow, your body and brain decay, and you age."

What can we do? "It starts with exercise," says Harry. "Exercise—the physical work of hunting and foraging—has always been the single most powerful signal we can send that life is good; that it's spring and time to grow."

"Biologically, there is no such thing as retirement, or even aging," Harry writes. "There is only growth or decay." And sedentary living, so common in modern times, is "the most important signal for decay."

Fortunately, we can swim against the tide for a very long time—if we chose to do so.

Exercise Signals Growth

Harry takes the reader inside the body for a look at how exercise affects the process of growth or decay. He says much of this is "new biology that has forever changed our thinking about aging."

I've heard that the body is constantly renewing itself, but I didn't appreciate the scale of the process. Every muscle cell in the body is replaced about every four months. "Your blood cells are replaced every three months, your platelets every ten days, your bones every couple of years." That's just scraping the surface, but you get the idea.

It's an active process. Your body doesn't wait for something to go wrong; it destroys and replaces the old parts on a natural schedule. Think of it as preemptive maintenance. "Biologists now believe that most cells in your body are designed to fall apart after relatively short life spans, partly to let you adapt to new circumstances and partly because older cells tend to get cancer."

If you exercise, each renewal is likely to be an improvement; if you don't, you may throw out more than you replace. Your muscles control growth or decay in the body. "The nerve impulse to contract a muscle also sends a tiny signal to build it up, creating a moment-to-moment chemical balance between growth and decay," not only in the muscle but throughout the body. "If enough of the growth signals are sent at once, they overwhelm the signals to atrophy, and your body turns on the machinery to build up the muscles, heart, capillaries, tendons, bones, joints, coordination, and so on."

"But let your muscles sit idle and decay takes over again."

Biology of Exercise

Your body was designed at a time when hunting and gathering was the way of life; it doesn't know any other way. Fortunately, it can't distinguish between walking in the park and foraging, or between jogging and hunting. The key is to understand that foraging and hunting have separate and distinct metabolisms. Sprinting and capturing wild prey are similar and involve a third distinct metabolism.

Light aerobic exercise (up to about 65% of maximum heart rate), walking and foraging, burns mostly fat for energy. It is "a wonderful pace," says Harry. "This is the metabolic zone where your body and brain heal and grow." Harder exercise builds more fitness, "but you gain more...general healthiness with prolonged light exercise."

Harder exercise (65% to 85% of max HR) is like shifting into second gear; you need more power than you can get from fat alone, so your muscles start to burn glucose. This shift is also "the signal that you've started to hunt."

Your ancient genes look on glucose as "powerful but expensive fuel," never to be wasted on foraging. "If you're burning glucose, you must be hunting, which triggers a major metabolic shift that affects your muscles, brain, gut, immune system, kidneys, liver, heart and lungs."

Finally, over 85% of heart rate capacity is anaerobic (without oxygen) exercise; it's like going into high gear. This degree of effort can only be sustained for a short time. It's reserved for "escape or capture" moments. "It saved your ancestor's lives, or let them end someone else's, countless times over the past few billion years." The modern equivalent would be the 200 meter dash, or Lance Armstrong sprinting for the finish line. Interval training, where the effort is hard, easy, and then hard again, uses high gear very effectively.

Anaerobic exercise is "great for vim, vigor and pure fitness," says Harry, but you need to "get into pretty good basic shape" before you try it. Preparation is required for those "escape or capture" moments. (See the "Warning" at the beginning of this book.)

(We'll talk more about energy systems in Chapter Five.)

Chris and Harry recommend that four days a week be devoted to aerobic exercise. That might be two days of light aerobics (walking) and two of medium to hard aerobics.

They, of course, recommend a total of six days a week of exercise: four days of endurance exercise—and two days of strength training.

Strength Training

Lifting weights until you can't do another rep forces your brain to activate the maximum number of strength units, nerve and muscle. It also damages the units, which is good, because it forces the body to rebuild them stronger and better than before.

That's why two days a week is enough for strength training. "Unlike endurance units, which recover from aerobic exercise overnight, your strength units need to enter a forty-eight-hour repair cycle [or longer]." (More about training frequency in the next chapter)

If you can handle them, free weights are better. Chris explains why: "They involve balancing and subtle corrections from side to side, all of which use and strengthen a whole bunch of other muscles and, more important, zillions of neuroconnections, which are at the heart of your ability to function in the real world."

Chris and Harry say everyone, especially those over 50, should be doing strength training. "Aerobic exercise saves your life; strength training makes it worth living."

(For more about Chris and Harry and their ideas on aging well, visit them online: www.youngernextyear.com.)

* * * *

While you're not likely to find "grow or decay" presented as a unified theory in an exercise physiology book—you'll remember that Harry pulled it together from many different sources—it's a logical framework to use when thinking about the many scientific studies showing the health-giving and anti-aging power of exercise (and leanness). Your exercise habits—your ability to walk, run, climb, lift, and play—are one of the most important determinants of how well and how long you will live. Let's talk about three of the most exciting recent studies.

Greater Fitness/Longer Life

Exercise capacity, your ability to consume oxygen and exert yourself, is perhaps the most powerful predictor of life span, a study published in the *New England Journal of Medicine* (March 14, 2002) concluded. The researchers found a direct relationship between fitness and survival.

As in other studies, the researchers found a "striking difference" in death rates between the bottom 25 percent in fitness and the next 25 percent. "This observation concurs with the consensus that the greatest health benefits are achieved by increasing physical activity among the least fit," the researchers wrote. They don't stress the desirability of becoming highly fit; they are more interested in encouraging people to begin exercising regularly. You've got to walk before you can run, of course; first things first.

Emphasizing the benefits of being very fit, as shown by the study, is my idea. I believe it's appropriate, because the study also found "a nearly linear [straight line] reduction in risk with increasing quintiles of fitness."

In my view, more people will continue exercising if they strive to be the best they can be. The greatest satisfaction comes when we continually challenge ourselves to improve. Progress makes training a lot more fun and rewarding; more than any other factor, progress motivates people to keep exercising.

See if you share my enthusiasm for the recent study. Here are a few of the details—and the bottom line conclusion.

The researchers found that each 1-MET increase in exercise capacity resulted in a 12 % improvement in survival. Participants whose exercise capacity was less than 5 METS were roughly twice as likely to die as those with exercise capacity of more than 8 METS.

METS or metabolic equivalents are a unit used to estimate the metabolic cost (oxygen consumption) of physical activity. One MET is the oxygen uptake when a person is at rest. Eight METS is the oxygen uptake running at six miles per hour.

Interestingly, absolute exercise capacity measured in METS predicted risk of death better than percentage of age predictions. (Not how fit you are "for your age," but how fit you are period.) What's more—get this—peak exercise capacity was found to be a stronger predictor of death than widely-known risk factors such as hypertension, diabetes, obesity, heart arrhythmia, high cholesterol, and even smoking.

In short, poor fitness proved to be the deadliest risk factor of all.

"No matter how we twisted it, exercise came out on top," lead author Jonathan Myers, a professor of medicine at Stanford University, told the *Washington Post*.

A truly remarkable study, I think you'll agree. Greater fitness means longer life. The fitter the better.

Fitness isn't everything, however. Leanness also matters.

Fit But Fat Risky

If you want to live a long and healthy life, fat but fit isn't the best way to go. Fit *and* lean improves your odds substantially more. Until recently, however, whether exercise can overcome the risk of being overweight has been controversial.

"There has been some suggestion that if you are particularly active, you don't have to worry about your bodyweight," said Dr. Frank Hu, lead author of a new study published December 23, 2004, *in The New England Journal of Medicine.* "That's very misleading."

The Harvard study was large and impressive, encompassing approximately 2.7 million person-years. The researchers followed 116,564 female registered nurses for 24 years. The nurses were 30 to 55 and healthy when the study began in 1976. The nurses, all non-smokers, were monitored for physical activity and body mass. The researchers found that being overweight or obese increased the risk of death regardless of the level of physical activity. Exercise helped, but did not overcome the higher risk of death associated with being fat.

Obese women who did brisk walking or other more rigorous activity three-and-one-half hours or more each week were, nevertheless, almost twice as likely to die as those who were both active and lean. Slender but inactive women were 55% more likely to die. Those who were both sedentary and obese were almost two and one-half times more likely to die.

"Women who were both lean and physically active had the lowest mortality," the researchers reported.

"Being physically active did not cancel out the increased mortality of overweight," Dr. Hu stated.

Clearly, the best way to live to a ripe old age is to watch what you eat *and* exercise.

Exercise not only extends our years, it improves the quality of the added years by improving our ability to learn and reason.

Aerobic Exercise Pumps Up Your Brain

We've had strong evidence for a long time that exercise brings blood and oxygen to the brain, resulting in improved mental function. A new study shows that exercise actually triggers measurable growth of brain volume in older adults, Arthur F. Kramer and Edward McAuley, researchers at the University of Illinois, Urbana, reported in the November 2006 *Journal of Gerontology*.

To appreciate the breakthrough nature of the new study and understand how rapidly our knowledge is growing, it helps to look back at an earlier study, published in the February 2003 *Journal of Gerontology*, in which Kramer and McAuley also participated.

The earlier study was the first to show (using high-resolution magnetic resonance imaging) significant differences in brain density between physically fit and inactive aging humans. "We found differences in three areas of the brain, the frontal, temporal and parietal cortexes," Kramer said in a news release. "There were very distinct differences particularly in two types of tissue, the gray matter and white matter." Nobody had reported this before, Kramer said at the time.

Gray matter consists of neurons and support cells that are involved in learning and memory, the news release explained. White matter contains nerve fibers that connect neurons throughout the brain. Older adults typically show a decline in both areas.

The 2003 study concluded: "These findings extend the scope of beneficial effects of aerobic exercise beyond cardiovascular health, and they suggest a strong solid biological basis for the benefits of exercise on the brain health of older adults."

The new study, published November 2006, goes further—it shows an actual reversal of brain loss.

Science columnist Sharon Begley wrote in *The Wall Street Journal* (November 16, 2006): "For the first time, scientists have found something that not only halts the brain shrinkage that starts in a person's 40s, especially in regions responsible for memory and higher cognition, but actually reverses it: aerobic exercise."

The details are explained in a University of Illinois release dated November 20, 2006.

Professors Kramer and McAuley, and their collaborators had 59 sedentary volunteers, age 60 through 79, do aerobic exercise (brisk walking), non-aerobic stretching and toning, or nothing for six months. The first two groups (aerobic and non-aerobic) started with 15 minutes of exercise and worked up to 45 minutes three times a week. Fitness was monitored and intensity increased as the study progressed.

High-resolution MRI was again used, this time to measure brain volume at the beginning and end of the six-month program. The stretchers-and-toners and the no-exercisers showed no change. The aerobic exercise group, however, showed a significant increase in brain volume.

"After only three months," Professor Kramer told the *WSJ*, "the people who exercised had the brain volume of people three years younger."

"This is a great emerging story," Fred Gage of the Salk Institute, La Jolla, CA, who led the 1998 discovery that humans can grow new brain cells, told the *WSJ*. "You can do something to influence your mental fate as you get older."

"You don't have to be a marathon runner—most people walk," Kramer said. "Swimming, biking and walking are all ways that people can get these anti-aging benefits."

Exciting stuff, huh? There are many more proven benefits of being lean and fit, but you get the idea.

Chris and Harry nailed it in *Younger Next Year*: Vegetate and decay, or exercise and grow. The choice is ours.

* * * *

The message of this chapter is simple and straightforward: If you're exercising, keep at it. If you're not, start now. Work up to six days a week, four aerobic exercise and two strength training. Your life and well-being may literally depend on it. Exercise for life.

Are you ready to discuss subjects that will help you get the most out the time you spend exercising? That's next. We'll talk about overload and the need for rest, the hotly debated issues of training frequency and slow lifting, and two important areas you don't hear much about: transfer of strength and balance.

"Stress. Recover. Improve. You'd think any damn fool could do it. But you don't. You work too hard and rest too little and get hurt."

Bill Bowerman
Bowerman, Kenny Moore, Rodale, 2006

Chapter Five

About Training

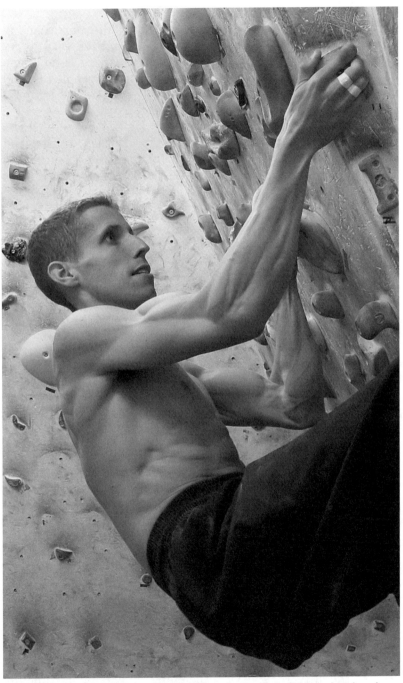

Jürgen Reis, world-class Austrian sport climber, doing what he does best. *Photo by Sebastian Nagel courtesy of Jürgen Reis*

Tower of Babel

Training is like building the Tower of Babel; there are so many conflicting voices telling you how to do it that it's easy to get confused. It's important to understand that there is no single *best way*. There are many ways that work. Some people respond better than others, but most reasonable methods of training produce results.

In his book, *The New Bodybuilding for Old-School Results* (Testosterone Publishing, 2006), Ellington Darden, PhD, asked celebrated bodybuilder Boyer Coe, "What's the most result producing arm routine you've ever experienced?" His answer is quite telling—and generally true for all body parts, and everyone.

"For me, anything that I did for my arms worked well," Boyer, who is known for his arm development, answered candidly. "One set to failure, super sets, pre-exhaustion, stage reps—fast or slow speeds—they all stimulated my arms."

That's a good thing. It means you have many options. When you tire of an exercise or routine, mentally or physically, you can generally renew enthusiasm—and restart progress—by moving on to something else. Change keeps you interested—and improving.

Overload and Rest

Some things never change, however. Don't lose sight of two basic requirements for productive exercise: overload and rest. Bill Bowerman, legendary Oregon track coach and co-founder of Nike, summed it up about as well as anyone could.

"Take a primitive organism, say a freshman. Make it lift, or jump or run. Let it rest. What happens? A little miracle. It gets a little better. It gets a little stronger or faster or more enduring. That's all training is. Stress. Recover. Improve. You'd think any damn fool could do it. But you don't. You work too hard and rest too little and get hurt." (*Bowerman* by Kenny Moore, Rodale, 2006.)

Overload is progressive stress. It simply says you must continually challenge yourself to do better. Do that, gradually and progressively, and you will become stronger and more enduring.

As Bowerman observed, most enthusiastic trainers "rest too little." That's the second requirement. You *must* give your body time to adapt to the demands of training.

"The body can be trained to greater performance by inducing stress," the late great George Sheehan wrote. "But the amount of stress and the time allowed for recovery are critical to the success of the process."

Overload and rest. Overload and rest. Overload and rest. Boiled down to its essence, that's what training is all about. Remember— and practice—both and your training will be successful.

(Sound oppressive and boring? Well, it can be. It can also be an endless adventure. Read on.)

Training Frequency

How does lifting twice a week sound? (That, of course, is what Harry and Chris recommend; but it's controversial.)

Arthur Jones, inventor of Nautilus weight training machines and founder of Nautilus Sports/Medical Industries, who recently passed away at 80, is widely known for his emphasis on brief and infrequent training. Probably more than anyone else in the weight training field, he stressed the importance of rest. Ell Darden's book, referred to above, alerted me to a review article on the validity of Jones' 30-year-old training recommendations. The survey of peer-reviewed literature by Dave Smith, PhD, and Steward Bruce-Low, PhD, both from the Department of Sport and Exercise Sciences at the University Liverpool in England, appears in the December 2004 Journal of Exercise Physiology (JEPonline).

The results probably came as a surprise to many exercise physiologists and coaches, who often disagree among themselves. Arthur Jones recommended training the whole body no more than twice a week; advanced individuals, he said, will often do better training only once a week. That's contrary to what we often hear and read.

"It is often suggested in the exercise physiology literature that novices train two or three times/week," Smith and Bruce-Low wrote, "but that more experienced trainees should engage in more frequent training." Some textbooks and groups call for split routines (training muscle groups separately) with four to six workouts a week, sometimes two or three times a day.

Jones went in the other direction. He said advanced trainees require more rest days, not less, to recover.

He wrote: "How many weekly workouts? Not more than two, and some people will produce better results from only one weekly workout. More is not always better, and in the case of exercise is usually worse."

Smith and Bruce-Low searched exercise physiology literature for studies dealing with training frequency. Given the time consuming nature of the advanced routines often recommended, they expected to find "at least [a] preponderance of scientific evidence" that high-frequency training produces better results than low frequency. Here's what they found.

Four studies show "no difference" in results from training once, twice or three times a week.

One study found that two or three times a week is "better" than once a week.

One showed that twice a week is better than three times.

One showed that three times a week is better than five times.

"Only" one study found more than three times a week "to be more effective."

Smith and Bruce-Low concluded: "For most individuals, training each muscle at most twice/week (and, in many instances not more than once/week) will provide optimal results." In short, the preponderance of peer-reviewed research, such as it is, suggests that Jones was correct.

(Smith and Bruce-Low also did a literature review on speed of movement, lifting slow or fast. We'll come back to that shortly.)

Bowerman's Heresy

The amount of rest required is also hotly debated in endurance training circles.

In *Bowerman,* Kenny Moore, a member of two Olympic teams (1968 & 1972) and former American record holder in the marathon with a time of 2:11:36, tells about the resistance, including his own, to Bowerman's theories on rest. In the August 2007 issue of *Runner's World*, Moore expanded the topic, including the experience of runners who came later.

Bowerman "sensed" that rest was as important as work "to keep a runner from illness or injury. If he erred, he wanted to err on the safe side of the cliff," Moore wrote. "His credo was that it was better to underdo than overdo."

This didn't go down so well with the coaching community. "When Bowerman first articulated the hard-easy method, he was widely despised for it," Moore relates. "The anthem of most coaches then was, *the more you put in, the more you get out.*" Coaches were "morally affronted. His easy days were derided... called coddling."

Moore adds parenthetically, "His common sense approach is still resisted by a minority, and probably always will be."

Bowerman's response was to "crush their runners with his." His "Men of Oregon" won four NCAA team titles. What's more, he coached 16 sub-four-minute milers at the University of Oregon.

Bowerman had to threaten Moore to make him listen to reason. "I was always sick or hurt," he wrote in *Runner's World*. "I was hewing to the promise that the more you put in, the more you get back. Can there be a bargain more just than that?"

"Finally fed up, Bowerman issued an edict. I was off the team unless I cut down my mileage and took easy days. This made all the difference. I stayed healthy, [and] made dramatic improvement."

"I owe my career of two Olympic Marathons to...Bill Bowerman," Moore declares.

Other runners weren't so lucky, Moore reports, citing as examples Todd Williams and Alberto Salazar.

"The finest American 10,000-meter runner of his era, Todd Williams, now admits to being 'psychotic' in preparing for the 2000 Olympic Marathon Trials. 'If the race went to the guy who trained with the hardest miles,' he swore, 'I couldn't lose.'

"And he still lost horribly; the miles reduced his tissues to catabolic soup."

Moore continues: "Alberto Salazar shortened his brilliant career and destroyed his health by doing such things as 100 hard miles the week after winning the New York City Marathon."

Moore quotes Salazar, "My coach at Oregon, Bill Dellinger, always told me not to overdo it. But when I disobeyed, he didn't call me on it. He let me get away with it."

The combined wisdom of Arthur Jones and Bill Bowerman says: More exercise is rarely the answer for a dedicated trainer, strength or endurance. More rest usually brings better results.

That's good enough for me. That's my experience.

Slow Lifting

I've never been a fan of slow lifting—until recently. (I'll explain my *partial* conversion in Chapter Eight.)

Let's see what Arthur Jones thought about speed of movement and whether the research literature agrees.

Some trainees insist on timing rep speed, taking as long as 10 seconds to raise the weight and 10 seconds to lower it. On the other extreme are those who use speed to cheat the weight up, taking about one-second or less to lift the weight and about the same to lower it. Both extremes are unpleasant and often dangerous. Lifting super slow can spike blood pressure and lifting fast can cause muscle pulls or worse.

(My friend Carl Miller, however, has been very successful teaching a momentum approach—based on the Olympic lifts—to all ages at his fitness center in Santa Fe, New Mexico. With careful supervision, fast lifting can be safe and effective. Olympic weightlifting, of course, by definition, involves fast lifting, producing perhaps the fastest moving athletes on earth.)

Most lifters are probably somewhere in between. They do what feels right, attempting to control the weight, up and down, and keep the stress mainly on the affected body part.

Arthur Jones recommended doing slow controlled reps, using a steady speed through the full range of motion. "Do not increase the speed as movement continues," Jones counseled. According to Darden, who worked with Jones for many years, this translates into about two seconds up and four seconds down. Jones didn't insist on timing rep speed.

Smith and Bruce-Low discovered that rep speed has been widely investigated. They found 20 relevant studies, including one involving cats. Some studies found that slow lifting increases muscle mass and strength significantly better than fast lifting. Others, however, examined fast (<2 seconds), intermediate (2-3 seconds), and slow (~6 seconds) rep speed and found no significant differences; all speeds produced about the same increases in strength. None apparently showed explosive lifting to be superior.

Overall, Smith and Bruce-Low found that studies "have tended to suggest that either slow training is superior...or that there is no difference between slow and fast speeds." They found no studies showing that lifting "at very fast speeds is superior for enhancing any aspect of muscle function."

Regarding Jones, they concluded that he was basically correct that "slow, controlled weight training is all that is necessary to enhance both muscle strength and power." It should be noted, however, that 2s up and 4s down, as Arthur recommended, is categorized by Smith and Bruce-Low as the *traditional* exercise speed. It's certainly not *super slow*.

(As I said at the beginning of this chapter, many methods work. I currently use both traditional and a form of slow lifting in my own training. I'll explain in Chapter Eight.)

Okay, but what about strength transfer? Is slow lifting (or fast lifting) better for certain sports? What's the best type of strength training to improve performance in specific activities or sports? The answer is straightforward and simple—once you understand the performance enhancement principles involved.

Transfer of Strength

I've always believed that a stronger athlete is a better athlete—in any sport. I remember reading years ago in one of Arthur Jones' *Nautilus Bulletins* that the best way to get stronger for a specific sport is to train the whole body in normal fashion. The worst thing you could do, Jones insisted, was try to mimic movements of the sport. For example, Arthur said that swinging a heavy baseball bat or golf club would be a mistake; it would only screw up your swing. Far better results would come, he said, from strengthening the total body with basic exercises, such as the squat, dead lift, bent-over row, bench press, and the overhead press—and then develop specific skills by practicing the sport.

Made sense to me; I believed it. But is it true? (Yes.)

Ellington Darden, mentioned earlier, began working with Arthur Jones in 1973, shortly after receiving his doctorate in exercise physiology from Florida State. He says the applicable principles of motor learning (movement skill acquisition) were well established at that time, but not well understood or even available to coaches and athletes. Arthur, however, understood the principles and, more importantly, their application.

"Jones reinforced to me," Darden writes, "in his unique way, that:

- "Strength training is general, requires overload, and best involves indifferent transfer.

- Skill training is specific, *requires no overload*, and best involves positive transfer.

- Activity that is *almost the same* as competition provides negative transfer, which complicates and wastes time." (Emphasis added)

That sums it up quite succinctly. The key is to distinguish between a general *ability* and a specific *skill*—and understand the three types of transfer: positive, negative, and indifferent.

Muscular strength is a general ability. It underlies a specific skill, such as swinging a baseball bat, hitting a golf ball, or kicking a football.

Studying motor learning has taught scientists that positive transfer results "when the activities of practice and competition are identical," Darden explains. When the practice is "almost the same" as actual competition, transfer is nearly always negative. "Almost-the-same activities cause the neuromuscular pathways to crisscross." Finally, when practice and competition are "totally unrelated" transfer will be indifferent.

One might think that indifferent transfer is useless and to be avoided, but as Arthur Jones reminded Darden, it can be a good thing—when it comes to general conditioning and strength training.

"It's the indifferent transfer of strength training that furnishes the stamina and conditioning necessary for the positive transfer from practice to competition," Darden writes. "That indifferent transfer of strength training combined with the positive transfer of practicing every movement of the game as it is to be played will assuredly lead to improved performance."

Richard A. Magill, PhD, a classmate of Darden's at Florida State University and the author of *Motor Learning and Control: Concepts and Applications* (McGraw-Hill, 8th Edition, 2007), confirms the motor learning concepts stated by Darden. (He does not specifically discuss strength transfer.)

"If a person's goal for learning to ride a bicycle is to deliver newspapers," Magill explains in his text, "then the greatest amount of transfer...will occur when the practice experience includes opportunities for throwing a newspaper while riding a bicycle." (This is positive transfer.)

Magill continues: "Negative transfer effects, which are typically temporary and overcome with practice, occur primarily when a new movement is required for a familiar environmental context."

As an example, he discusses why golfers don't always transfer their performance on the practice range to their play on the golf course. Condensing and paraphrasing the lengthy explanation in the textbook, he says they don't practice like they play. Among other things, they don't practice the types of situations they would expect to experience during an actual round of golf. With more actual competitive experience, however, they may eventually be able to incorporate more of the skills learned on the practice range into their game. Negative transfer, he says, can often be resolved in time.

No real surprises there, except perhaps the reference to the temporary nature of negative transfer. Note, however, that Arthur Jones said activities that are "almost the same" produce negative transfer, which "complicates and *wastes time.*" No one wants to complicate the effects of training unnecessarily and waste time, right?

Magill does add a few new wrinkles, but they're basically technicalities and don't really change the practical considerations.

Bottom line: Forget running with ankle weights, performing exercises on unstable surfaces and similar *almost the same* activities. Stick to standard weight training exercises—and practice your sport.

That brings us to balance, an important subject rarely discussed in books such as this.

Balance

No matter how old we are or how active we may be, we can all benefit from exercises or activities that improve balance. Balance is important in all sports and the physical activities of daily life. While age is a factor, lack of practice/exercise can contribute to balance problems at any age.

Here's a simple way to assess your balancing ability.

According to *RealAge.com*, how long you can stand on one leg with your eyes closed without losing your balance is an indication of your functional age. My friend and former doctor at the Cooper Clinic, Arnie Jensen, always had me to do this as part of my physical exam.

RealAge says 15 seconds is very good if you are 45 or older. The average time a 60-year-old can remain steady on one leg with eyes closed is 7 seconds; by age 70 it drops to 4 seconds. At the other end, the average for someone in the 25-to-30 age range is 28 seconds.

It's another case of use it or lose it. Most people don't exercise their balancing skills as they age and, as a consequence, their eyes, ears, muscles, brain, and nerves progressively lose the ability to keep them upright.

I like to practice balancing when I'm washing and putting away my dishes in the morning. It makes a mundane activity fun. I start by balancing on one leg and then the other with my eyes open. And then, after I'm finished with the dishes, I try it with my eyes closed, while standing in front of the sink to spot myself.

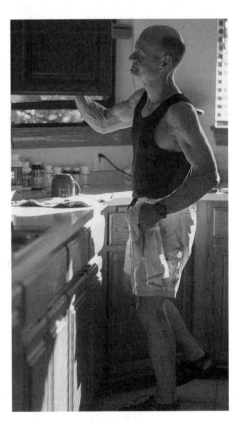

Look carefully at the photo, and you'll see that I'm balancing on my left foot while putting my dishes in the cabinet. When I close my eyes, it's a whole new ballgame. *Photo by Laszlo Bencze*

I've worked up to 20 seconds with my eyes closed, but not without practice. Some days I'm pretty good at it, and other days not so good. Either way, it turns doing the dishes into a little game. Believe it or not, I actually look forward to doing the dishes.

Regular weight workouts also help to maintain and improve balance. As Chris Crowley pointed out in *Younger Next Year*, free weights—barbells and dumbbells—are better than machines for this purpose. "They involve balancing and subtle corrections from side to side," Chris says, "all of which use and strengthen a whole bunch of other muscles and, more important, zillions of neuroconnections, which are at the heart of your ability to function in the real world."

The mention of neuroconnections made me wonder what Professor Magill says about balance. What I found is interesting and useful.

First, Magill says there is some dispute among researchers whether balance is a general ability or a combination of many specific skills. It appears that it's both. As you'll recall from our discussion above, abilities are best trained generally and skills specifically. Balance should probably be trained both ways.

Balance is usually thought of as static or dynamic. Both seem to be relatively specific. Being good at one doesn't necessarily mean you'll be good at the other. As we'll see, you need to practice both.

Static balance, which refers to the maintaining of equilibrium while in a stationary position, is·considered to be a simpler variation of dynamic balance, which refers to maintaining of equilibrium while in motion. With this in mind, many rehab protocols undertake to develop static balance skills before moving on to dynamic activities, such as walking—which certainly seems logical.

The problem, however, says Magill, is that "evidence consistently indicates that static and dynamic balance are relatively independent motor abilities."

"At the most basic level," says Magill, "we need to consider static balance and dynamic balance as two independent types of balancing ability. Beyond that," he continues, "we need to view the ability commonly called 'balance' as specific to the task or skill in which balance is involved."

It seems pretty clear that we should practice both static and dynamic balance. In addition, we should practice specific skills in which we want or need to improve.

My balancing game at the sink is mostly static, although moving around on one foot and then the other, while washing, drying, and putting away the dishes, adds a little dynamism; it makes it more fun as well.

Another dynamic balance I've had fun with is the heel-to-toe walk. We've all heard about it being used in field sobriety tests. You simply position your heel just in front of the toe of the opposite foot each time you take a step; your heel and toes should touch or almost touch with each step. You can make it more interesting by changing the pace and direction, fast or slow, straight or in circles, right or left. If you want to make it really exciting, try closing your eyes.

Walking on irregular surfaces also challenges dynamic balance. Carol and I enjoy hiking on the many trails in the foothills above our home. We can make it as challenging as we want.

Most forms of exercise—walking, running, biking, swimming, strength training—help improve balancing ability. The key is to do many forms of exercise, including some specifically for balance. And keep doing it!

* * * *

This chapter focused on matters not usually covered in books on training. We talked about progressive overload and the necessity of rest; training frequency (it's better to underdo than to overdo, in both weights and aerobics); lifting speed (both slow and fast work, but not too slow or too fast); strength transfer (make the whole body stronger, and then practice your specific sport); and finally, balance (it's important and should be trained specifically).

What about diet (not dieting)? That's next.

"You don't need to be a scientific investigator to eat right, constantly counting milligrams or calculating percentages. It simply involves keeping the emphasis on the whole foods available on the perimeter of the supermarket rather than on the boxed, bagged, canned, and other packaged goods lining all the center aisles."

> Miriam E. Nelson, PhD, and Alice H. Lichtenstein, DSc
> *Strong Women, Strong Hearts*, Putnam 2005

Healthy eating is not a black-and-white proposition; it's about eating the right foods most of the time.

Chapter Six

About Diet (Not Dieting)

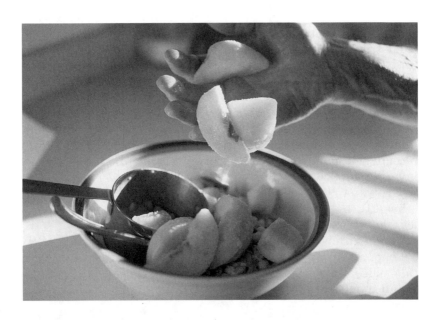

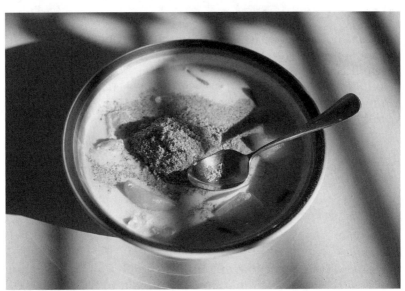

Photos by Laszlo Bencze

The Secret

It seems that people are always looking for the magic bullet. They love "quick fix" diets. As a result, they resist or ignore the real secret: Severe or unbalanced diets provide temporary results at best. In the long-run they just don't work.

It's true that some bodybuilders use extreme diets to get into contest shape. They cut their carbohydrate intake to practically nothing, they adopt very low fat diets, try to live on mostly protein, or flat-out starve themselves. Top female models apparently do the same thing at times. The body simply can't function properly for long on such diets. If you saw many bodybuilders a few weeks or months after a contest, you probably wouldn't recognize him or her. That's because extreme dieting is almost invariably followed by bingeing.

The way to look—and feel—your best is regular exercise and a healthy, balanced diet containing enough calories to provide for your energy needs day in and day out.

The next few sections will look to two very wise and practical experts for an overview of healthy eating. After that, we'll talk more about the importance of the essential fats (omega 3 and omega 6) and several other things that I believe will interest you.

Healthy Eating Patterns

No one does a better job explaining complex health matters in an easy-to-understand way than Tufts University professor and researcher Miriam Nelson, author of the *Strong Women* book series. Nelson's primary expertise is in physical activity, and she teams up with authorities in other areas to write about a wide variety of health and fitness issues. Her book *Strong Women, Strong Hearts* (Putnam 2005), written in collaboration with Tufts' nutrition and cardiovascular-disease expert Alice H. Lichtenstein, DSc, includes the clearest explanation I've seen on how women (and men) should eat to avoid heart disease and generally stay healthy. What follows draws heavily from their chapter entitled: Don't Think Diet—Think Food Patterns.

Vegetables and Fruits

Healthy eating starts with lots of vegetables and fruits. Four or five servings of vegetables and two to four of fruits is a good goal. Carol and I don't count servings, but we have one or both with almost every meal and snack. We use both fresh and frozen produce. Carol likes to buy in-season produce; she peels, slices, dices and (if necessary) cooks, from scratch. I like the year-round convenience of the frozen food department, which offers up every imaginable variety and combination of produce, frozen at the peak of freshness, and ready to eat after thawing. We always have a bowl of fresh fruit—usually apples, but it could be any fruit in season—on the counter in the kitchen and sliced carrots or other ready-to-eat vegetables in the refrigerator; fruit and vegetables are our default snacks at any time of the day or night.

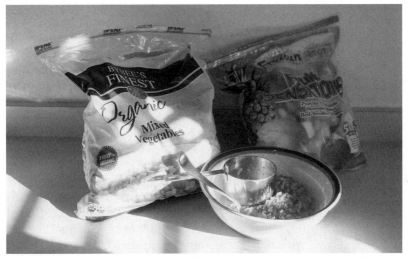

Supermarkets everywhere are filled with wonderful frozen fruit and vegetable mixtures. Look for those with nothing added—no sugar or sauce—just fruit and vegetables. *Photo by Laszlo Bencze*

What's so special about vegetables and fruits? For starters, produce is high in fiber and bulk, and low in calories. It's also high in potassium and very low in sodium, both of which help keep your blood pressure low. (High potassium and low sodium also improve muscle definition.) Moreover, Nelson and Lichtenstein say there is a remarkable "consistency" in the studies showing that diets rich in vegetables and fruits are "associated with a decreased risk for developing heart disease and stroke." The truth is that vegetables and fruits are filling without being fattening—and just plain good for you.

Carol and I almost never drink fruit or vegetable juice, however. Professors Nelson and Lichtenstein explain why: "Whole fruit [or vegetables], unlike juice, offers fiber. And it tends to be more filling. An orange will stave off mid-morning hunger much better than a glass of orange juice." Whole produce makes you feel full and satisfied, without giving you too many calories. It takes up room in your stomach that might otherwise be filled with fat-and-sugar-laden foods.

No discussion of produce would be complete without a word or two about the much-maligned potato. "Potatoes are decent vegetables that have been unfairly criticized," Nelson and Lichtenstein write. "Their skin is a decent source of fiber, and the fleshy part contains lots of potassium and a reasonable amount of vitamin C, along with other nutrients."

Potatoes are starchier than other vegetables, and they do contain more carbs. "Think of potatoes as a grain rather than a vegetable," the Tufts professors suggest. "That is, they're not instead of broccoli; they're instead of bread, rice, or pasta."

Carol and I often share a big baked potato with our dinner, but almost never with butter or sour cream; balsamic vinegar or non-fat yogurt is our favorite topping. Needless to say, we almost never eat French fries, which are loaded with salt and extra calories—and, according to Nelson and Lichtenstein, often contain trans-fatty acids because of the fat in which they are fried. We steer clear of potato chips for the same reasons.

Any kind of plain, unembellished vegetable or fruit is good. A wide variety is best. Try to include several different colors in each meal: green, red, yellow—make your plate look like a rainbow. For example, sliced carrots and a few cherries or slices of watermelon go well with a nut-butter sandwich at lunch. Broccoli, sweet potato, and a green salad with tomatoes enhance any dinner. Use your imagination and you can't go wrong.

The Right Fats

The idea is to replace most unhealthy fats with healthy fats—and not eat too many calories in the process. "[Unhealthy fat] includes the saturated fat in beef, poultry, and other meat as well as full-fat dairy foods, and the trans-fatty acids in commercially fried and baked foods and other items, including the legions of packaged foods that run the gamut from cookies, cakes, and crackers to microwavable popcorn and frozen entrees," the Tufts professors write. That doesn't mean you can never eat a juicy T-bone or filet mignon or chocolate cake, just that such indulgences should be infrequent. Healthy eating is not a black-and-white proposition; it's about eating the right foods most of the time.

Nelson and Lichtenstein say low-fat diets are out and moderate-fat diets are in—"as long as you have the right fats." Those include the polyunsaturated fatty acids in fish, seeds, nuts, and many vegetable oils. Conventional wisdom says that oils high in monounsaturated fatty acids, such as olive oil and canola oil, are exceptionally healthy. "The scientific evidence no longer supports that line of thinking," Nelson and Lichtenstein report. Monounsaturated oils are good for us, but not uniquely so. "The [primary] aim is simply to shoot for more unsaturated fat and less saturated and trans fats."

Carol uses some olive oil in cooking and on salads. I have a teaspoon of canola oil in my coffee at breakfast and before workouts. Other than that we prefer to get most of our fats from whole foods. We have fish several times a week (more on that later); we also have ground flaxseeds—in my breakfast cereal and in her morning smoothie. I have a nut-butter sandwich most days (more on that, too), and Carol likes walnuts.

We are careful about how much total fat we eat.

A gram of fat contains nine calories, compared to four in protein and carbohydrate. Too much fat is still fattening. The idea is to replace bad fat with good fat, not pile on good fat. We don't count calories, but calories do count, especially fat calories, which are easily converted to body fat. Overloading with fat of any kind will make you fat, so be careful.

Whole Grains

Carbohydrates, the major component of grains, have been blamed for our ever-expanding waistlines. "It's not so," Nelson and Lichtenstein state emphatically. "Carbohydrates are GOOD FOR YOU."

Refined carbohydrates are a problem, however. Sugar and white flour are two of the purest forms of refined carbohydrates; all the fiber and bulk have been removed, leaving nothing but concentrated—and empty—calories. Sugar is the main component in soda pop, and sugar and white flour are the main ingredients in white bread, pizza dough, and pretzels. Compound the problem by adding butter or lard to make cakes, cookies, and the like, and you're really in trouble. Refined-grain foods will add calories to your diet and inches to your body. Plus, they lack vital nutrients needed to keep you healthy.

The good grains are whole grains, such as those found in whole-grain breads and cereals, brown rice, and whole-wheat pasta. "Unlike refined grains, they contain fiber plus a host of nutrients and healthful plant chemicals that are eliminated when grains go through the refining process," the professors explain.

Whole-grain foods are sometimes hard to identify, however. The no-brainers are whole grains available in natural food markets and many traditional supermarkets. These are the intact, unbroken grains as they come from the field; examples are oat groats, rye, barley, millet, spelt, kamut, amaranth and many others. Whole grains can be cooked like rice and served plain or take the place of pasta. Carol and I use whole grains as breakfast cereal or in place of rice at lunch or dinner.

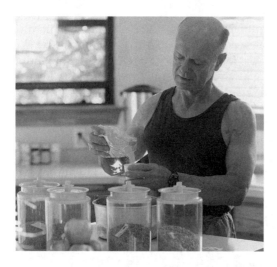

You'll find a wide variety of whole grains at health food markets and many regular supermarkets. Carol and I store ours in canisters kept in a cabinet made for that purpose. (Note the apples on the counter.) *Photo by Laszlo Bencze*

After the intact grains, it gets more complicated. "Only 5 percent of the packaged grain-based products in the supermarket are whole grain," the co-authors warn. "And it's not easy to tell which ones they are." Terms such as multi-grain, seven-grain, and unbleached don't tell you whether the grain is whole. The magic word is "whole" and it must be part of the first ingredient on the label to insure that the food contains whole grain. Brown rice means whole-grain rice is in the package. Popcorn is also whole grain. "Make sure it's air-popped rather than made with butter or partially hydrogenated fat (trans-fatty acids)," Nelson and her colleague caution.

About the only packaged grain product Carol and I use regularly is bread. We like the whole and sprouted grain breads made by Food For Life, which are now widely available. Our favorite is Ezekiel 4:9 Sesame, a sprouted grain bread (more tips on choosing bread later in this chapter).

Four to nine servings of grain products are recommended, at least half from whole grains. Half would be an improvement for most Americans, but more would be better. Almost all the grain products Carol and I eat are whole grain. Again we don't count servings, but I have grains three or four times a day, usually in the form of intact grains, bread, or oatmeal. (Some oats are more refined than others, but all forms contain the whole-grain components: groats, rolled, steel-cut and oatmeal. Instant oats are best avoided, however, because they find their way into the blood stream too fast.)

Low- and Nonfat Dairy Foods

"Diary products are associated with stronger bones and may keep down blood pressure," Nelson and Lichtenstein write. They are, of course, an excellent form of complete protein, calcium, and other nutrients. The downside is the saturated fat they contain, so it's important to select the low- or nonfat form. I always buy nonfat dairy foods, usually skim milk or nonfat yogurt. Being a little more adventurous, Carol sometimes goes for low-fat cheese or cottage cheese. Low-lactose varieties are available for those who have trouble digesting dairy products. Soymilk is also an acceptable substitute for milk and other dairy foods (not for babies, however). I alternate soymilk and skim milk.

I use skim milk (or unsweetened soymilk) on my breakfast grains, and nonfat yogurt as a topping for fruits, vegetables, and baked potatoes. Nonfat yogurt is an extremely versatile food and goes with just about anything.

Two to three servings of nonfat dairy foods are recommended. I often have more than that, but some authorities question whether that's a good idea. Walter C. Willett, MD, chairman of the Department of Nutrition at Harvard School of Public Health, believes dairy may have a dark side. "A diet high in dairy products has been implicated as a risk factor for prostate cancer," Willett wrote in *Eat, Drink, and Be Healthy* (Simon & Schuster 2001). Surprisingly, saturated fat isn't the troublemaker; it is a problem, of course, but doesn't seem to be the cancer connection. "Calcium might be the culprit," Willett opines. Here's the doctor's plausible explanation: "Inside the prostate (and elsewhere), the active form of vitamin D may act like a brake on the growth and division of cancer cells. Too much calcium slows or even stops the conversion of inactive vitamin D to its biologically active form and so may rob the body of a natural anticancer mechanism."

This is far from settled—Nelson and Lichtenstein do not cite a possible cancer connection—but it's something to keep in mind. Moderation is almost always a good idea, even when it comes to something as innocuous and wholesome as diary products.

Healthy Proteins

We've mentioned dairy products as a good source of protein, but there are many excellent sources. A wide range of protein containing foods is probably best, not all at once, of course, but over time. Nelson and Lichtenstein list fish, beans, soy, eggs, nuts, skinless poultry, and lean forms of beef, pork, and lamb. Get your protein from a variety of sources, but don't overdo it. Most Americans eat more protein than they need, often the wrong kind. Twenty percent of calories is about right; hard-training athletes can probably benefit from as much as 25 percent. Have at least one source of high-quality protein with each meal and you'll be fine. Three or four servings daily are recommended.

Saturated fat, again, is a problem. The professors suggest proteins that don't come packed with a lot of saturated fat. Fish should be near the top of the list. "The evidence is overwhelming that including fish in the diet helps stave off heart disease," the authors write. They suggest at least two fish meals a week.

Fish high in omega-3 fatty acids, such as salmon (wild is best), sardines, herring, mackerel, and other fish with darker-colored flesh are good for your heart. (See below) "But we don't want you to get hung up on the type of fish you eat," they state. Vary the type of fish you eat, and almost any fish that suits your taste is fine. "Your risk of mercury toxicity or toxicity of other contaminants [PCBs] is quite low," says Doctor Lichtenstein. Remember that she suggests eating a variety of fish, and only a few times a week. (For small children and women of childbearing age, check Food and Drug Administration guidelines for restricted species, which are very few.)

With a few limited exceptions, any fish is good for you. "Even tuna sandwiches count—but fish sticks, fried clams, and fried, breaded shrimp do not." The method of cooking is important. Baked or broiled is best. Deep-fried is a no-no, however, because of added calories and often trans or saturated fatty acids. Carol sometimes adds flour and seasoning and cooks fish in the skillet with a little olive oil (works for chicken too). She usually bakes or broils our fish, however.

Beans are often overlooked as a protein source. Uniquely, beans are relatively low calorie—and contain lots of fiber and essentially no saturated fat. Canned beans are the most convenient. Look for brands with little or no added sugar and fat. Ideally, what you want is beans, and nothing else. The international section of your supermarket is a good place to look; we buy a Mexican brand that's simply beans and a little added salt. "Throw them into tossed salads, add to vegetable stir-fries and to your favorite soups, or simply have them as a side dish," the doctors suggest. Tofu fits into much the same category—high in protein and practically no saturated fat. It can be used in many of the same ways.

"Beef, pork, and chicken are fine on our heart healthy plan, too, especially if you broil or grill them," the Tufts professors write. The key is to buy the leanest cuts of meat and skinless chicken— and "keep the portions on the small side." It's not exactly the American way, but think of chicken and meat as a side dish, not the main course. It works great for Carol and me. It gives us the wonderful flavors and complementary protein, while keeping calories and saturated fat low.

And don't overlook the high-quality protein in eggs. Moderation, again, is the key. Yes, eggs are high in cholesterol, but that's not as much of a problem as once thought. "We now know that while the cholesterol in food can raise blood cholesterol, saturated fat and trans-fatty acids generally raise blood cholesterol—and heart disease risk—considerably more," the Tufts experts relate. "The amount of cholesterol in your food doesn't correlate with the amount of cholesterol in your bloodstream."

Dietary cholesterol is still important, but three or four eggs a week are fine—especially if the rest of your diet is relatively low in cholesterol. Or you can have more eggs, and discard half the yokes. The important thing is the total amount of cholesterol in your diet. Keep in mind that all animal-based proteins (meat, fish, dairy) contain some cholesterol.

With cholesterol as well as the other components we've been discussing, it's the overall balance that counts. Remember: lots of fruit and vegetables, unsaturated fat, whole grains, low- or nonfat dairy, and lean protein.

Pick up a copy of *Strong Women, Strong Hearts* at your local bookstore or on Amazon.com. Man or woman, you'll be glad you did. What I like about the dietary advice in this book is that it doesn't confuse the reader with a lot of complicated and questionable rules. Nelson and Lichtenstein give you the fundamental facts, and don't sweat the small stuff.

Now, as promised earlier, let's talk about the omega fats, 3 (found in fish, flax, and green leafy vegetables) and 6 (which is rarely a problem). It's a fascinating tale, one that's only now coming into focus.

The Omega Problem

What is the "omega problem," and why is it important?

"The problem [is] that the tissues of Western populations [are] awash in omega-6s, fats that compete with the omega-3s," Susan Allport writes in *The Queen of Fats*, (cited in Chapter Three). In her excellent book, published in 2006, Allport tells how we discovered that consuming too much of one essential fat and not enough of the other is a problem.

Let's start with a brief look at a recent study that quantifies the dangers presented by contaminants in fish and clearly establishes the connection between fish and heart health.

Harvard researchers analyzed years of data and concluded that the health benefits of eating fish far exceed the potential risks from contaminants. They determined that the cardiovascular health benefits of wild-salmon consumption, for example, outweigh the cancer risks by 900 to one, while the benefit of farm-raised salmon outweigh the risk by 300 to one. The Harvard review, published October 18, 2006, in the *Journal of the American Medical Association*, found that people who eat one or two servings of fish per week, especially fatty varieties such as salmon, may reduce their risk of death from heart attack by 36% and overall death rates by 17%.

Science writer Allport tracks the long and winding road that brought us to the conclusions made by the Harvard researchers—it's a detective story of epic proportions. I've always liked fish. My dad, a medical doctor, was a great fly fisherman, and loved eating his catch. (Carol doesn't care for the taste of fish.) None of us, however, had the slightest inkling of the uniqueness of the fat in fish. After hearing the details, you'll want to join Carol and me in eating fish regularly.

I won't tell the whole story here, you can read Allport's book for that, but I will give you what appear to be the high points. They are fascinating—and demonstrate how the scientific process works. It's more hit or miss than we sometimes think.

It starts in the 1970s when Danish physicians Hans Olaf Bang and Jorn Dyerberg went to Greenland to investigate Eskimos who ate large amounts of seal and whale blubber, without suffering from heart disease. Fat, of course, was thought to be "the dietary demon that causes this disease."

Mystery Fat Discovered

Bang and Dyerberg collected the blood of 130 Eskimos, who lived by fishing and hunting. Among other things, the doctors wanted to know if their blood lipids would match their high fat consumption.

Tests on the spot showed that the Eskimos had low levels of all of the lipoproteins, except HDL. (The specimens were then frozen and taken back to Denmark for further testing.) "This outcome was not surprising, given the Eskimo's low incidence of heart disease, but it was surprising in light of their diet rich in animal fat and cholesterol," Allport explains. "Moreover, it seemed to be the result of dietary rather than genetic differences, since Eskimos living in Denmark had lipid profiles resembling those of Danes."

Their paper in the journal *Lancet* reporting these findings (a mere curiosity when published) has since become a nutrition classic—mainly because it was the first to record high levels of HDL-cholesterol, now known as "good cholesterol," in people with a low incidence of heart disease.

Even more important, in the view of Allport and others, was their suggestion that the explanation was "probably the large amount of polyunsaturated fatty acids in the fat tissue of the animals eaten [lot of whale and seal blubber]."

The Danish researchers went on to analyze the 130 frozen samples they had brought back from Greenland to determine the basic building blocks of the lipids in the Eskimos' blood. Comparing the lipid make-up to that of Danes, they found "a striking difference in the two populations," Allport writes.

The Eskimo blood contained a very small amount of arachidonic acid—an offspring of linoleic acid, the only fat known at the time to be essential for human health—and a very large amount of a fatty acid they were unable to identify. "The Eskimos had seven times as much of this mystery fat as did Danes, and about one-seventh the amount of arachidonic acid."

Determined to identify the mystery fat, Dyerberg flew to the United States to consult with Ralph Holman, a world authority on the composition and function of fats. Holman quickly identified the substance as eicosapentaenoic acid (EPA), and a smaller amount of another fatty acid known as docosahexaenoic acid (DHA), which was also present in larger amounts in Eskimos than in Danes.

Dyerberg left Holman's lab knowing that eicosapentaenoic acid (EPA) was important, but it took another chapter in the mystery to determine how important. This time the key player was Ralph Holman. (To give you a hint, arachidonic acid is a member of the omega-6 family, and EPA and DHA belong to the omega-3 family.)

New View on Fats

This episode starts with the tragic death of Ralph Holman's mother. She was hospitalized for a condition that destroyed her bowels in the early days of intravenous feeding. Fat being insoluble in water, the first intravenous solutions were fat free.

As noted early, linoleic acid was known to be essential for human health; it could not be produced internally and had to be provided in the diet. Holman suspected that other fatty acids might be essential as well. "His mother's doctor was receptive to what Holman was telling him about fatty acids (as many doctors at the time were not)," Allport relates, "but neither of them could figure out how to safely provide her with the nutrients she was missing."

When the next life-or-death situation came along, informed by the work of Bang and Dyerberg with Eskimos and other developments, Holman was ready.

In 1979, Holman was asked to consult in the case of a six-year-old girl, who had been accidentally shot in the stomach. "The wound...would make her the first human case of omega-3 deficiency ever to be recorded in the scientific literature," Allport writes.

Much of the girl's intestine and colon were removed, and she had to be fed intravenously. Unlike the case of Ralph's mother, linoleic acid (omega 6) was included in the IV. She did well for almost a year, but "then she began having episodes of tingling, numbing, and weakness in her legs, sometimes accompanied by blurred vision and a total inability to walk," Allport relates. "It was a peculiar array of symptoms that the neurologists treating her had never seen before."

Fortunately, one of her physicians, Terry Hatch, suspected that her intravenous nutrition might be the problem. Ralph Holman was called in to do a fatty acid analysis of the girl's blood.

Holman found that she was deficient in omega-3 fatty acids and also that her intravenous preparation was very low in omega-3. He suggested that she be switched to a preparation "based on soybean oil and containing both linoleic and alpha linolenic acids (in a ratio of 6 to 1)," Allport relates. "In twelve weeks, all of her neurological symptoms had disappeared."

Alpha linolenic acid, ALA, is the parent of the omega-3 family and the precursor of EPA and DHA, which Bang and Dyerberg found in abundance in the blood of Eskimos.

Dr. Hatch, who in 1982 joined with Holman to publish their findings about the young gunshot victim in the *American Journal of Clinical Nutrition*, told Allport he didn't think the case "made a lot of impact." Nevertheless, Allport writes, "For Holman and a few other researchers, [the girl's] case brought a sea change in attitudes, a new way of looking at the world." It meant that omega-3 deficiency could impact, perhaps cause, heart disease and neurological disorders, even obesity (see Chapter Three).

Fish-Oil Cure

The medical community's reaction to the young girl's case was essentially, "So what?" The case was looked on as an aberration. "What does it matter if alpha linolenic acid is essential for humans, when it is almost impossible to make someone deficient?" is how Allport describes the reaction.

Holman was not deterred, however. The case suggested to him that the "fat that Dyerberg and Bang had brought to the world's attention should be thought of as a nutrient whose absence was helping to *cause* heart disease." Unable to impact the medical community in a meaningful way, he began "proselytizing" to his friends—with some pretty amazing results.

When a colleague, Dale Jarvis, was home on disability leave after bypass surgery, Holman suggested that he start taking fish oil. "He became one of the first people to take massive doses of fish oil to correct a heart problem, a treatment now widely recommended," Allport relates.

"Within a few days," Allport reports, "Jarvis was up and pushing his lawn mower" and within weeks was back at work. All the while, Holman was checking his blood and found that his omega 3s, which were low at first, "soon jumped to four times that of controls."

Jarvis had more than two decades of good health before having a second bypass operation.

That apparently put us on the long road to the 2006 Harvard-study recommendation: EAT FISH. As noted earlier in Chapter Three, Allport also recommends eating lots of fruits and vegetables. Again, she says green vegetables are "full of alpha linolenic acid, the parent omega-3 fatty acid." Stick to the "good" fats described earlier in this chapter, and be sure to include fatty fish.

For many more fascinating and convincing details, read Susan Allport's *The Queen of Fats*. (In case you're wondering, omega-6 fats are the king, because they were the first to be found essential to human health.)

On a less serious note (with an omega fats connection), I promised more about my long-time favorite, the peanut sandwich. Believe it or not, peanut butter has been improved.

New Peanut Butter!

New peanut butter? Yes. The first big innovation since "all-natural" peanut butter came on the market about 15 years ago: more and better protein, less fat, and fewer calories, more good fat—and better taste. That's exciting for a guy who made his bones, so to speak, by reducing his body fat to 2.4% eating peanut butter sandwiches for lunch.

Peanut butter was introduced to America in 1890, as a protein supplement for people with poor teeth who couldn't chew meat. The next step in the evolution of this enormously popular food—1.25 billion jars were consumed in 2003—wasn't until 1922, when a California entrepreneur formulated peanut butter with a yearlong shelf life. (Ouch, I'm not sure that's a good idea nutritionally.)

That was it until PowerButter, a 15-year-old Alabama company, introduced two high-protein, essential-fatty-acid fortified, natural peanut butters: *Peanut PowerButter*™ developed for the health-food-store/athlete market and *Naturally More*™ for the mass market. (The latter is my favorite: fewer calories, great taste and less expensive.)

Perfect Protein

The first hurdle was figuring out how to enhance the incomplete protein in peanut butter (three essential amino acids are low), without ruining the creamy consistency and terrific taste. The simplest solution turned out to be the best: add pasteurized egg white.

In addition to neutral taste and proper consistency, egg white contains all nine essential amino acids and a usability rating of 94%—compared to 85% for milk and only 74% for beef. Importantly, egg protein has a surplus of the three amino acids lacking in peanut butter.

The result was impressive: 32 grams of protein in PowerButter, compared to only 14 in a 4-tbsp serving of regular peanut butter. *Naturally More*™ has slightly less protein, 20 grams in a double serving (serving size: 2 tbsp.). Remember, too, that the protein in both products is almost totally useable, while only 50% of the protein in regular peanut butter is functional.

Essential Fats

The fat in peanut butter, mostly monounsaturated, is not so much good as not bad. So the next big idea was to fix that by adding essential fatty acids in the form of flaxseed and flax oil. As explained earlier, most of us consume more than enough omega-6, but are low on omega-3, where flaxseed and flax oil shine. By removing most of the peanut oil and replacing it with flaxseed and flax oil, PowerButter raised the percentage of omega-3 fat to 37% and lowered omega-6 to 10%, compared to 0% and 29%, respectively, in regular peanut butter. (Flax oil is a less efficient source of essential fats than fish, but fish oil wouldn't exactly be a taste-enhancer.)

The net result of adding egg white, flaxseed oil, and fiber-rich flaxseed (along with a few other ingredients) is a substantial reduction in total fat, 20 grams compared to 32 in peanut butter. And fewer total calories: 364 in PowerButter and 338 in

Naturally More™, compared to about 400 calories in the same amount of regular peanut butter.

Great Taste

As an experienced consumer of peanut butter, I can say that both products are creamier and taste better than plain (natural) peanut butter, which tends to be a bit dry and hard to spread. One of the secrets is the addition of dextrose (sugar) in PowerButter and honey in *Naturally More*™. It must not be much, however, because there are only 6 grams of sugar in PowerButter and 4 in the same amount of *Naturally More*™.

The only downside I see in the PowerButter products is added sodium, 260 mg versus zero in raw peanut. That's an acceptable trade off in an otherwise low sodium diet—unless you are salt sensitive.

Why Peanut Butter?

Some of you, especially new readers, may be wondering why a guy interested in lifetime leanness would eat calorie-dense nut butter. The answer is simple and lies at the very core of my diet philosophy.

I like nut butter, and it's a bad idea to deprive yourself of foods you enjoy. That doesn't mean you should gorge on high-calorie foods such as nut butter. You should allow yourself such foods in measured amounts. That's what I do.

Diets based on denial are psychologically flawed. As I wrote in *Ripped 3*, "It's human nature to crave what you can't have, and craving usually spells doom for dieters." I don't have cravings—because I don't deny myself foods such as nut butter.

Carol and I are not the only ones who like these new peanut butters. PowerButter is available at GNC and *Naturally More*™ is available at Wal-Mart and Wild Oats (which recently merged with Whole Foods). Other stores have these products as well, of course, more all the time; ask where you shop.

In case you're wondering, we have no financial interest in either product.

Now, as promised, let's talk about shopping for bread.

The Art of Choosing Bread

Tara Parker-Pope explained the problem not long ago in *The Wall Street Journal, Health Journal*: "The supermarket bread aisle is packed with hearty-sounding multi-grain and wheat varieties. But many of them aren't much more than dressed up white bread."

Choosing good bread is trickier than you might think. Here's my solution.

As explained previously, bread is good for us, provided it's the right kind. Eaten as part of a balanced diet, it's not fattening. I eat bread every day. The problem is that the white bread most people eat has the bran and germ stripped away. Without fiber, bread is quickly absorbed, causing a spike in blood sugar, which gives you a burst of energy followed by a crash soon after.

Like Professors Nelson and Lichtenstein, Parker-Pope suggests checking the label. "The presence of whole grain makes all the difference," she says. The first ingredient should include the word "whole." Check the label for fiber content as well. One gram or less of fiber per slice is a red light. Three grams of fiber is a good sign.

You're still not there, however.

Armed with these tips, Carol and I went to the supermarket. After carefully examining the breads available, we bought one clearly labeled "Whole Grain Nutrition" and "100% Whole Wheat." The first ingredient listed on the label was "stone ground whole wheat flour." Each slice contained 3g of fiber. As icing on the cake, the USDA Food Guide Pyramid was depicted on the wrapper, with the "Bread Group" at the base. It looked like a good choice. The check-list items were all there.

When we got home and tried it, however, we were disappointed. The bread was soft and airy, with no structure; it literally melted in your mouth. What's more, it left an unpleasant aftertaste. To us, it was refined bread. It certainly wasn't our idea of good bread. It met the requirements. Still, it was not good.

Apparently, "whole grain" doesn't make *all the difference*. Something was missing. This is where the art of bread selection comes into play.

Weight Matters

We compared the bread we had purchased with Sprouted Grain Ezekiel 4:9 Sesame, a firm, full-bodied, chewy bread made by Food for Life—and my favorite. Surprisingly, both loaves weighed the same (24 oz.). The slices were noticeably different, however.

One slice of the "100% Whole Grain" bread weighed 28g, while a slice of Ezekiel weighed 34g—21% more.

Weight matters. It explains why the Ezekiel is so dense and chewy. It's also why the other bread is so soft and airy—and no doubt quick to digest.

When selecting bread, check the weight on the label, but don't stop there. Pick it up and squeeze it. Good bread, such as Ezekiel, will be firm. Compare it with a loaf of white bread. The difference will be obvious. White bread and many of the "stone ground," "cracked wheat," and "multi-grain" breads—even some of the "whole grain" breads—will be light and squishy. Put them back on the shelf.

The Ezekiel bread also has more calories per slice, 80 versus 60 for the other bread. But that's not necessarily a bad thing. "Giving up calories can mean giving up fiber," Tara Parker-Pope warned in the WSJ.

The sprouted grains in the Ezekiel bread are well worth the extra calories.

Sprouted Grain Bread

Sprouted grain bread has no flour, which is a major advantage.

The milling process used to make flour cracks the grain and separates the endosperm from the bran and germ. The endosperm is then ground to the desired consistency to produce the final product. For whole grain flour, the bran and germ are returned at the end of the process. White flour consists of only the ground endosperm. Because of the presence of bran, whole grain flour is higher in fiber and naturally heavier and denser than white flour. Both types of flour, however, consist of relatively small particles—and are quickly absorbed into the blood stream.

Here's why: "As particle size decreases, G-Force [glycemic or blood sugar impact] generally increases," Nikki & David Goldbeck explain in *The Healthiest Diet in the World* (Plume, 2001). "For example, the G-Force of wheat kernels increases as you go from the whole berry, to cracked wheat or bulgur, to more finely ground couscous, and finally to flour."

That's why we chose sprouted grain bread over bread made with flour. The particle size of the sprouted grains in Ezekiel bread is clearly larger than the particles in bread made with flour, white or whole-grain. Again, compare Ezekiel bread to bread made with flour. Look at both carefully and break them up. The particles in the Ezekiel bread are clearly larger. Put the Ezekiel bread in your mouth and chew it; feel the structure and graininess. As the Ezekiel bread label says, "Your body and taste buds will know the difference!"

Bread made with sprouted grains is chewier and more satisfying than bread made with flour. It stays with you longer.

(No, we don't have a financial interest in Food For Life Baking Company either.)

As we've noted, bread is mostly carbohydrate, and carbs are good for us. That's especially true for active people and athletes, the type of person likely to be reading this book.

Facts on Carbs for Active People

Carol and I are fans and admirers of Lance Armstrong as a seven-time winner of the Tour de France and an inspiration and advocate for people battling cancer. Lance's longtime personal coach, Chris Carmichael, has written a book on nutrition. *Carmichael's Food for Fitness* (Putnam, 2004), written with Jim Rutberg and Kathy Zawadzki, is unique in that it's not about losing weight or preventing some life-threatening disease. *Publishers Weekly* says it's written for "a minority group living in a society struggling to cope with serious health issues," namely athletes and active people. An excellent book, it explains in straightforward, easy-to-understand language the how and why of eating to fuel an active, performance-oriented lifestyle.

Carmichael agrees that athletes and active people need plenty of carbs. "While low-carb diets have their merits for a select population," he writes, "a nutrition program higher in carbohydrates is much more appropriate for you as an athlete."

Why becomes clear in his discussion of intensity and fat burn, and low-carb diets.

Intensity and Fat Burn

Having written about the so-called fat burn zone (see Chapter 3), I was eager to learn Carmichael's take on the topic. "It's important to realize that you burn carbohydrates, protein, and fat simultaneously whenever you exercise, regardless of the intensity," Carmichael writes. "There's no such thing as an exercise that only burns fat." The proportions do change with the intensity of the exercise, however.

As briefly noted in Chapter 4, three primary energy systems are involved every time you exercise—immediate, aerobic (with oxygen) and anaerobic (without oxygen)—and the percentage of energy supplied by each system shifts as the intensity of the workout changes. Your diet and fitness level also influence the energy source.

The immediate energy system isn't a major energy supplier, because it can only supply energy for about 8 to 15 seconds. The aerobic and anaerobic systems are the main producers.

At low intensity, 20 to 25 percent of maximum effort, most of the energy is supplied by fat, from food and mobilization of fat stores. "It's important to note, however, that in order for your muscles to burn fat in the aerobic system, carbohydrate has to be present," Carmichael explains. "In conditions where your body is depleted of carbohydrates, the rate at which you burn fat decreases, and your capacity for high-intensity disappears."

At 40 to 50 percent of maximum effort, you burn roughly 50/50 fat and carbs, almost all through the aerobic system. "The percentage of energy derived from carbohydrate increases as intensity increases, in part because you need energy more quickly than it can be liberated from fat," Carmichael continues. "If it were possible to only burn fat for energy, you would be limited to exercise under 60 percent of your maximum effort."

The shift to burning more carbs than fat occurs when the anaerobic system comes into play. "Fat can only be oxidized through aerobic metabolism, but carbohydrate is burned aerobically and anaerobically," writes Carmichael. When the aerobic system can no longer keep up with increasing intensity, the anaerobic system kicks in and fat-burn percentage goes down. The relative contribution from carbs, on the other hand, increases with the intensity.

From 50 to 85 percent intensity, the contribution from fat continues going down. The aerobic system is still providing a large portion of the energy, however. Above 85 percent, the proportion of energy from fat decreases even more.

Hmmm. Sounds like the fat-burn-zone crowd may be onto something. But wait.

"You're still burning a lot of fat," Carmichael assures readers. "You may derive the highest percentage of your energy from fat when you exercise at low aerobic intensities, but when you increase your intensity, *you burn more total calories and more fat.*" (Emphasis added)

Finally, Carmichael adds another fundamental point, one that I made earlier: "Low intensity exercise is also less likely to induce enough of a training load to improve fitness." To become more fit, you need overload—and carbs. Greater fitness enables you to do more work aerobically and anaerobically—and burn more fat.

As you've probably figured out by now, the energy systems are also central to the low-carb issue.

Low-carb Diets

Chris Carmichael: "Low-carbohydrate diets were devised to help overweight and obese people lose body mass in order to improve health. They were not devised with the intention of improving performance." To the contrary, such diets inhibit athletic performance.

As noted, high intensity exercise is impossible without adequate carbohydrates; fat simply cannot supply energy fast enough to support maximum performance. That doesn't mean low-carb diets have no merit, however. "Considering the fact that low-intensity exercise can be beneficial for primarily sedentary people and that low-intensity exercise may be sustainable on a low-carb diet," Carmichael reasons, "sedentary people may benefit from low-carb diets." That's not true for active people and athletes, however.

The basic idea of the low-carb diet is that depriving the body of carbohydrates will force it to burn fat. As low-carb dieters know, this is called ketosis. In the absence of carbohydrates, your body transports fatty acids to the liver to be converted to ketone bodies. Ketones provide the brain and central nervous system with the steady supply of energy required for survival. Carmichael warns, however: "You can't generate energy anaerobically with ketones, which is one of the reasons *athletes on low-carbohydrate diets struggle to sustain even moderate-intensity exercise.*" (Emphasis added)

This explains bonking or hitting the wall, which usually occurs when blood sugar starts running low. Glucose (blood sugar) is the preferred fuel for your brain and central nervous system. "Bonking is your body's way of forcing you to stop exercising while there is still enough glucose in your blood to maintain normal bodily function," Carmichael writes. "Athletes eating low-carbohydrate diets bonk earlier than normal because they start workouts glycogen-depleted. As a result, they have far less fuel than needed to supply energy for muscles and the central nervous system."

* * * *

We'll end this chapter with a sobering—and empowering—thought: "Even one meal of a double cheeseburger with fries and a Coke will mess up your system, let alone a steady diet of it, which is a recipe for disaster." (Cardiologist James O'Keefe, MD, Mid America Heart Institute, Kansas City) The next two sections are about two studies that illustrate the magnitude of the problem and provide a solution available to practically everyone.

Every Meal Counts

A surprising new study at the Heart Research Institute in Sydney, Australia, has made me think again about the three or four desserts I often enjoy at family gatherings on major holidays. The study shows what saturated fat does to your arteries—and it ain't pretty.

The study led by Dr. Stephen J. Nicholls, a cardiologist now at the well-known Cleveland Clinic, is straightforward in design and carries a powerful message. It's reported in the August 15, 2006, issue of the *Journal of the American College of Cardiology*.

Fourteen healthy subjects were fed two meals separated by one month. The meals were equal in calories, with one gram of fat per kilo of body weight. The difference was in the nature of the fat. One meal was high in unsaturated fat (75% polyunsaturated, 10% monounsaturated, and 9% saturated), and the other high in saturated fat (90% saturated, 6% monounsaturated, and 2% polyunsaturated).

Again, all subjects consumed both meals, a month apart.

Saturated fat, as explained earlier, is generally thought to be unhealthy, and poly- and monounsaturated fat healthy. "Fatty acid composition has a profound impact on the influence that dietary fat exerts on cardiovascular risk," the researchers note.

In plain language, they undertook to find out how each meal influenced the stickiness of molecules produced by the cells that line blood vessels, and how that influences the flow of blood in the arteries and veins. They wanted to know how the two types of fat help or hinder HDL cholesterol in protecting against clogged arteries.

They looked at artery function at three points in times: before and 3 and 6 hours after each meal. Bypassing much of the medical jargon, here's what they found.

First, HDL cholesterol collected after the saturated fat meal was accompanied by a higher level of adhesion [sticky] molecules expressed [squeezed out] by artery wall cells. In contrast, HDL cholesterol collected after the unsaturated-fat meal was accompanied by a significantly lower level of sticky molecules. Importantly, the level of sticky molecules at both 3 and 6 hours after the unsaturated-fat meal were *lower than before the meal.*

My interpretation: After a meal high in saturated fat, the blood is more likely to clump and stick to the artery wall, impairing blood flow. On the other hand, a meal high in unsaturated fat may actually improve the ability of arteries to accommodate blood flow.

Dr. Nicholls and his colleagues concluded: "Consumption of a saturated fat reduces the anti-inflammatory activity of HDL, and impairs arterial endothelial [lining] function. In contrast, the anti-inflammatory activity of HDL improves after consumption of polyunsaturated fat."

The eye-opener is that the effect of a high fat meal is immediate. I certainly didn't know that, and I'll bet you didn't either. I thought artery blockage happened over a long period of time. That's true, it does, but it can also occur in a split second.

James O'Keefe, MD, a cardiologist at Mid America Heart Institute in Kansas City, got to the heart of the matter: "When you eat the wrong types of food, inflammation and damage to the vessels happens immediately afterwards."

I believe one dessert will be enough for me at the next family gathering.

Moreover, I'll be sure to exercise later in the day. The next study shows why.

Exercise Counters High-Fat Meal

I have often tried to walk off the bloated logy feeling after a high-fat meal. It always makes me feel better, but does exercise actually have a measurable effect on artery function? Does it counter the negative effect of a high-fat meal shown in the Australian study?

Doctoral candidate Jaume Padilla and his colleagues at the Departments Kinesiology Nutrition and Medicine at Indiana University, Bloomington, proved that it does indeed. Their study is reported in the September 2006 issue of the *European Journal of Applied Physiology*.

Exercise not only works, it makes artery function better than before the high-fat meal.

They subjected eight healthy individuals to three treatment conditions administered 2 to 7 days apart: 1) Low-fat meal alone (LFM), 2) High-fat meal alone (HFM), and 3) High-fat meal followed two hours later by aerobic exercise (HFM+EX).

Both meals contained about 940 calories. The high-fat meal included eggs, sausage, and hash browns; it contained 48 grams of fat (16.5 saturated and 4.5 trans fat). The low-fat meal included cereal with skimmed milk and orange juice; it contained no fat.

The subjects walked on a treadmill for 45 minutes at 60% of their measured VO2peak. They rated the intensity "fairly light" to "somewhat hard"—so we're talking about a relatively comfortable pace.

Here's the researcher's bottom-line conclusion: "These findings suggest that a single aerobic exercise session cannot only counteract the postprandial [after meal] endothelial dysfunction induced by ingestion of a high-fat meal, but also increase brachial artery [flow] in apparently healthy adults."

Simply put, artery function was better after exercise than before the meals. Almost sounds like you can have your cake and eat it too—if you exercise. (Well, almost)

Words to the Wise

This study is part of a growing interest in the direct effect food has on the body. An online press release from Media Relations at Indiana University states: "After a fatty meal, arteries lose their ability to expand in response to an increase in blood flow, with the effect peaking four to six hours after eating—just in time for the next meal." It seems that many of us are eating in a manner that impairs artery function virtually around the clock. That can't be good, and it's not.

"What happens four hours after that high-fat meal is that your artery looks just like the arteries of a person who has heart disease," said co-author Janet P. Wallace, a professor in the IU Department of Kinesiology. "What our study shows is that when you exercise after that meal, it doesn't look like a sick artery anymore."

The problem, of course, is that no one wants to exercise after every meal. If you eat healthy foods, as recommended earlier in this chapter, you won't have to.

As shown in the first study, the type of fat is also important. One can't help wonder what the result would've been had Padilla and his colleagues included a fourth treatment condition combining exercise and a meal high in unsaturated fat. Would artery function four hours later have been even better? Sounds like a pretty good bet, doesn't it?

Bottom line: Eat smart—and exercise.

* * * *

This chapter suggested broad guidelines—not hard and fast rules—for every-day healthy eating. Vegetables and fruits, the right fats, whole grains, low- or nonfat dairy foods, and lean protein are all part of a healthy diet. We tracked how omega-3 fatty acids were discovered to be essential and learned that they protect against heart attack and prolong life. I told you about a new and improved peanut butter, and we talked about choosing good bread. We looked to Lance Armstrong's coach for a detailed explanation of why active people and athletes need carbs. Finally, we discussed a study showing how a high-fat meal impairs blood flow and another showing how exercise helps your blood flow freely.

Next, let's talk about using this information to achieve and maintain top condition. I'll tell you what I eat normally and the changes I made to get ready for the photos you see on these pages.

There's no need to eat foods you don't like—even when peaking—and there's no need to ever leave the table feeling hungry.

Chapter Seven

Eating for the Peak

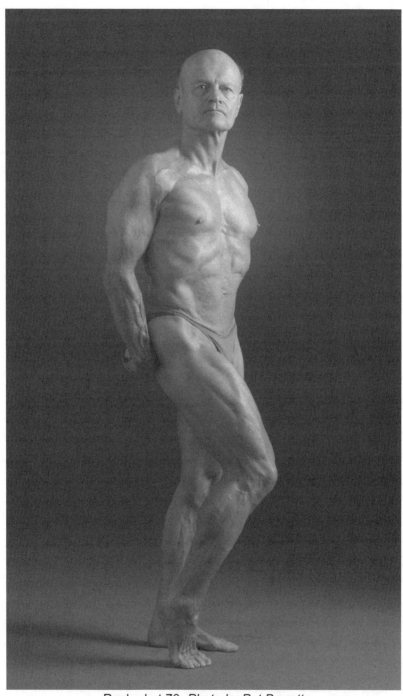
Peaked at 70. *Photo by Pat Berrett*

Dieting Philosophy

My dieting philosophy is that I don't believe in dieting. I don't diet in the normal sense of the word, ever, even when peaking.

The word "dieting" gives the wrong impression; it has an unpleasant connotation. I use it here only to distinguish between what we talked about in the last chapter, healthy eating patterns, and what we will be discussing here. This chapter is about eating to achieve peak condition for photos, a contest, a class reunion, or any time you want to look your best, which is different, a little more controlled. Not as different or controlled as you may expect, however.

"Dieting" conjures up thoughts of hunger and deprivation. Dieting doesn't work, because it makes people uncomfortable and unhappy. I believe the key to permanent body fat control is eating satisfaction. There's no need to eat foods you don't like—even when peaking—and there's no need to ever leave the table feeling hungry.

That doesn't mean there's no discipline involved. There is. It takes effort and planning to achieve peak condition. If you eat the right things at the right time, you can eat as much as you "really" want—and still create a slight negative calorie balance. Eating slightly less than you burn is all that's necessary. Do that consistently and your fat cells will notice the calorie deficit, but you won't. If you feel tired and hungry or deprived, you've gone over the line. You should feel good.

The key is to eat foods that make you feel full and satisfied, without giving you too many calories.

The foods that do that best are whole foods, the way they come in nature—with little, if anything, added or subtracted. That means lots of vegetables and fruit, whole grains, low- or nonfat dairy foods, small amounts of chicken and lean meat, and some fatty fish—the same foods we talked about in the last chapter. The only difference when training for peak condition is that you need to be more consistent and careful about what and how much you eat. (I will tell you what I eat, meal by meal.)

And one more thing—very important: Don't skip meals. Stay ahead of your hunger curve. Come to each meal under control. It's okay to be a little hungry, but not ravenous. Eating regular meals is a key factor. It keeps you in the frame of mind to stay on plan—and increases your odds of success tremendously.

If you screw up occasionally, don't worry about it. Consider it a lesson learned and resolve to do better next meal. What you eat most of the time is what's really important. Make it a point to stay satisfied, however, and you will rarely be tempted to stray—I promise.

I start the peaking process by making a careful assessment of my condition. You can't map out the best way to your destination until you know where you are.

Keeping Track

I don't count calories or anything else in my diet, but I do monitor changes in my body. I keep track all the time, but I pay more attention when I'm preparing for photos. I don't enter physique contests any more, but I do compete with myself. I take photos periodically to compare my condition from year to year. Photos are how I keep track long term. The mirror and body composition measurement are how I do it from day to day and week to week.

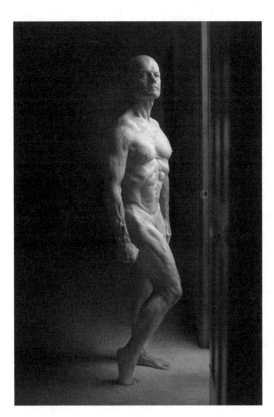

Every morning when I get out of bed, I look at myself in the mirror just before putting on my clothes. There's nothing like looking at your nude body to assess your condition. If you don't like what you see, it motivates you to do something about it. If you're satisfied with your progress, it's a great way to start your day. Either way, it's a real eye-opener. *Photo by Laszlo Bencze*

In addition to using the mirror, I urge you to buy a body composition scale to monitor what's happening to your body. That gives you an objective measure of how you are doing. Changes occur very slowly and are hard to detect when you see yourself every day. Having an outside measure that gives it to you straight provides an early warning (or confirmation), and allows you to make small course corrections as required. I'll tell you how I do it.

I weigh on my Tanita Body Composition Scale every Saturday morning before breakfast—and record the result. The original Tanita scale that I started using in the late 1990s shows bodyweight and body fat percentage. It was (and is) a wonderful boon to the record keeping I started decades ago; it makes it much more convenient to track changes accurately. I no longer have the expense and hassle of having myself weighed underwater from time to time.

The new model that we purchased early in 2006 gives many more readings. It gives more information, but also makes the whole process more complex. If you don't understand how the readings are generated, it can be confusing and perhaps a bit off-putting.

The key to using body composition measurements is to realize that all methods are educated guesses or estimates—none of them are absolutely accurate. All body composition tests use a set of assumptions, which vary from method to method; the assumptions may or may not fit your situation. Accept the tests for what they are—and do not expect absolute accuracy.

Most tests do a good (not perfect) job of tracking change in response to diet and exercise—and that should be your focus. All tests, however, without exception, will give consistent results *only if you use them consistently*. To get consistent results, you must be consistent; you must weigh under the same circumstances every time.

As noted, I weigh before breakfast on Saturday morning. It's okay to weigh on a different day or at a different time, as long as you are consistent from week to week. If you weigh on Tuesday evening before going to bed, then you must weigh at that time every week. (As I will explain shortly, evening readings are usually lower than early morning readings; expect your body fat to be one or two percent lower in the evening. That doesn't mean you will look better, however; you may look more defined in the morning when you are *slightly* dehydrated. Too much water loss, however, will make you look flat.)

New and Improved Monitors

In addition to bodyweight and fat percentage, the new scales measure—estimate—total body water, visceral fat, muscle mass, bone mass, and daily calorie expenditure. Body weight and fat percentage are probably adequate for most purposes, but I've found value in the additional measurements—especially body water percentage or hydration level, which has a major effect on the body fat and muscle mass readings.

When hydration goes up, so does the muscle mass reading. That's because muscle is about 70% water. Fat percentage, on the other hand, goes down, which is also logical. More muscle generally means less fat.

That explains why your fat-percentage reading is likely to be lower in the evening. We all tend to be dehydrated in the morning, after going all night without water and empting the bladder upon arising. Body composition, of course, hasn't changed in any meaningful way from morning to evening. That's important to know when tracking change in response to diet and training. It also illustrates why accuracy requires that you weigh at the same time every week.

Another change is that the new monitor asks for your age, along with height, sex, and whether you are an athlete; the old monitor didn't consider age in the body fat calculation. The literature that comes with the new scale explains why age was added. I don't buy it, however, at least for someone like me who has worked hard to maintain or improve overall body composition. Tanita seems to concede this point in their literature.

"Research has determined that as we age there is a tendency to increase body fat [especially visceral fat] and decrease muscle mass," says Tanita. My fat readings over the last nine years show that that did not happen in my case. "This is a natural progression," says Tanita, "unless you increase exercise as you age." That's probably correct. I believe, however, that training intensity is what matters most, not volume. I have not increased volume, but I have maintained training intensity—and I didn't gain fat or lose muscle over the last nine years. My first and last fat percentage readings on the old scale, as well as the average of the first 10 readings and the last 10, are almost exactly the same.

To evaluate how age affects the readings on the new scale, I weighed myself using both the default age (30) and my actual age at the time (68). The fat percentage and muscle mass were the same on both age settings. When my actual age is entered, however, Tanita's proprietary formula moved part of the fat to my belly. On a scale of 1-59, my visceral fat rating is "1" on the default setting, and "7" using my actual age. Both ratings are *healthy*, according to Tanita; 1 to 12 is healthy and 13 and above indicates an excess level of visceral fat.

For the average person, however, especially those who have not been training, I suggest using your actual age—and not changing it over time. That way you'll know what's actually happening. If you change the age setting every year, you'll be accepting, as a fact of life, that you *will* get fatter with each passing year, at least in the belly. (As explained in Chapter 3, there is no physiological reason to gain fat with age. The choice is yours.)

The new Tanita literature also does a better job explaining the "Athlete" mode. On both the old and new models, you are offered a choice of Male or Female or Male/*Athlete* or Female/*Athlete*. If you select *Athlete*, you are automatically given the highest setting for *activity* (another new feature), which means you are involved in intense physical activity.

Tanita defines *Athlete* as someone who exercises for at least 10 hours a week and has a resting heart rate of 60 or lower, which is basically the same as before. But they've expanded the category to include "lifetime of fitness" individuals who've been fit for years but "currently exercise less than 10 hours per week." They also specify that it does not include "enthusiastic beginners," whose bodies have not had time to change sufficiently to require the Athlete mode for accuracy.

"Athletic body types are physiologically different than standard adult body types," Tanita explains, "due to muscle mass and hydration differences. Athletes generally have greater muscle mass and *tend to be more _dehydrated_. These differences would skew [an athlete's] body fat reading high, when taken with the standard Adult mode."

As I recall, the dehydration factor wasn't explained in such detail when our first scale was purchased. Hydration is very important, because the basic assumption of Bioelectrical Electrical Impedance (BIA), the method used by Tanita scales (old and new), is that "lean muscle has more water than fat tissue and allows the [electrical] signal to pass more easily." Fat causes more "impedance" or resistance than muscle. That means the Adult mode short-changes athletes on muscle mass two ways. First, it assumes less muscle (and more fat) than athletes typically have, and second, it compounds the error by interpreting dehydration as a permanent muscle deficiency, rather than a variable condition. That's why I usually suggest that most people, especially active trainers, use the Athlete mode from the beginning, and stick with it. That will give a more accurate initial reading—and show changes in response to diet and training.

In addition, Tanita apparently assumes that body water level decreases with age. When I enter my actual age, the new scale calculates my total body water at 60 percent or slightly higher; using the default age (30) it's almost 70 percent. It's unclear what the formula does with the decrease in water when I enter my actual age. As noted above, my muscle mass (given in pounds) and fat percentage are the same on both age-settings.

As I said at the beginning of our discussion on keeping track, I encourage everyone to buy a body composition monitor (made by Tanita or other manufacturers). Get one with all the bells and whistles. Don't obsess over the new information, however; use what applies to you and helps you achieve your goals, and ignore or discount the rest. Remember that body weight and fat are still the most important variables for tracking your progress.

Buy the best monitor your pocketbook allows. And read all the literature that comes with it. The more you understand about how your scale works, the happier you will be.

My Readings

One might think my body composition readings are not as helpful as they could be, because I believe in staying lean year-round. There's some truth in that, because the changes in my body composition will not be as dramatic as they would be if I had a lot of fat to lose. The process is the same, however, for everyone. My example, however, may be especially instructive for those approaching maximum leanness.

As I write this (early May 2007), I've been in peaking mode for about nine months. On July 22, 2006, I wrote in my training diary: "Carrying some fat on my sides and lower back—going to start paring fat down slowly. Want to sharpen up abs for photos later this year or early next. I'll start by simple being a little more careful each meal." That's essentially the "dieting philosophy" explained at the beginning of this chapter.

It worked, but there was a bit of a problem. As I recounted in chapter two, a stricture developed in the neck of my bladder following my earlier surgery, and repeat surgery was required to remove the restriction. That made my body composition record look like a roller coaster.

I started weighing 156.4 pounds with 6.2% fat. The next week I was 154.8 and 7.5%, respectively, for a two week average of about 7% fat. That's my starting point.

Fourteen weeks later, after consistent "dieting" and training (the only workouts I missed were when I was in the hospital), and corrective surgery, I bottomed out at 146.4 pounds and 5% fat. Unfortunately, I lost about 5.5 pounds of muscle in the process.

The muscle loss was not good (medical problems curbed my appetite and forced me to train with less intensity), but the 2% fat loss was quite good for someone already at 7%.

Losing 2% fat in 14 weeks sounds pretty slow. Why is that good? Because losing faster is likely to trigger ancient survival mechanisms that favor fat over muscle; the body thinks a famine is coming, and prepares by storing extra fat. Fat is the body's most concentrated form of energy, and the best guarantee of survival when food is scarce.

Severe dieting (or starvation) causes the body to produce more of the enzymes responsible for depositing fat. These fat-depositing enzymes create a tendency to get fat. Severe dieting also causes a slowdown in metabolism.

This isn't just a theory. It has happened to me on several occasions. Cutting calories too severely caused me to lose weight *but gain fat*. On one occasion, I lost 5.6 pounds, and my body fat went up. I lost a little over 6 pounds of muscle and *gained* a pound of fat. Not good!

It's important to take your time shedding fat, when you are already relatively lean—or any time. As we just explained, your body interprets rapidly decreased weight as a threat to survival. As a general rule, don't try to lose more than one pound a week; one half pound is probably safer and more sustainable. Losing faster makes you uncomfortable and inclined to binge—and might even cause you to gain fat. Your long-term success in reducing body fat, whether or not you're shooting for a competitive level of leanness, will depend largely on your patience. Don't rush the process.

Considering my medical setback, losing roughly 3.5 pounds of fat was good. Regular exercise gave me a major edge over the average sedentary individual. My guess is that many people in similar circumstances would have lost muscle, and gained fat.

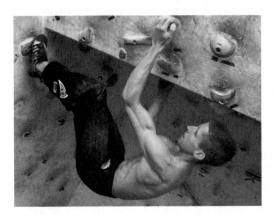

Pure muscle and bone is what's needed to do this.

Photo by Sebastian Nagel courtesy of Jürgen Reis

Be that as it may, my job at that point was to stay lean and gain back the lost muscle—and that's what I did.

With 24 weeks of consistent eating and good training (and a perfectly functioning bladder), I regained about 5 pounds of muscle (varied from week to week) and kept my body fat around 5% (or lower). That's where I am now, about seven weeks away from the main photo shoot for this book.

As an aside, which may or may not be true, I suspect that my new Tanita scale is not programmed to go below 5%. I say that because the scale has repeatedly given me 5% readings, but never lower. At the same time, my old model Tanita scale has registered 3.5% a number of times recently. Interestingly, when Austrian sports climber Jürgen Reis (www.juergenreis.com) visited with us early in 2007, our old model Tanita showed his body fat to be 1.5%. I know that sounds incredible, but he looks to be pure muscle and bone—not an ounce of fat visible anywhere. The new Tanita showed him at 5% fat.

Now let's move on to what I actually ate.

Meal Modifications

I will describe each meal, and then explain the changes made to create a calorie deficit and start my body fat on a slow downward path. My meals were already balanced and healthy, and my

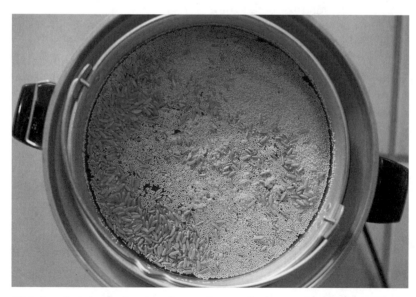

This is a batch of mixed grains and water in the cooker; it's enough for about 10 days. Cooking is automatic and takes about 2 hours. Store in refrigerator after cooking. *Photo by Laszlo Bencze*

weight was stable. A little tweaking was all that was necessary, enough to get the attention of my fat cells—without making me uncomfortable.

These meals are good, but not magic. Neither are the specific modifications. The meals and the changes are simply examples of my dieting philosophy in action. What I'd like you to focus on is the unhurried and moderate nature of the changes.

Let's start with breakfast. I'll list what I normally eat—and then explain the changes.

Breakfast

1 double-sized mug of coffee (two-thirds skimmed milk, 1/3 water, one packet Sweet'n Low, and one teaspoon canola oil)

Cereal mixture:

1 cup mixed whole grains (oat groats, hulled barley, spelt, kamut, and amaranth prepared every 10 days or so in a Tatung Automatic Cooker & Steamer: 6 cups mixed grains and 18 cups water)

1 handful frozen mixed vegetables (carrots, corn, green beans, and peas)

1 handful frozen mixed fruit (peaches, pineapple, honeydew melon, seedless grapes)

1 cup Silk plain unsweetened soymilk

2 tablespoons flaxseed, ground

2 teaspoons Splenda no calorie sweetener (optional)

(*Microwave 5 minutes*)

The modifications, I know, will seem almost inconsequential. That's the point. Over time, taken with other small adjustments made during the course of day, they will have a meaningful impact.

Let's start with the coffee. I like the big mug (holds over 2 cups), but I used more water (and less milk), and I only filled the cup about two-thirds.

In the cereal, I usually use a heaping cup of the cooked grains; I cut back to a little less than a full cup. Likewise, I usually fudge a little on the mixed vegetables and mixed fruit, throwing in a *little more* than a handful. I dropped back to one handful of each, and no more. I also backed off to a little less than a cup of soymilk. Finally, I cut back to one tablespoon of flaxseed. (All small changes, but they add up.)

Mid-Morning Snack

Wild salmon, canned (about a quarter cup)
1 medium apple

Every other day or so, I substitute a cup of plain unsweetened soymilk for the salmon, which drops about 30 calories. An apple is filling and goes well with just about anything.

Lunch

Naturally More™ peanut butter sandwich with 2 slices Eziekiel 4:9 Sprouted Grain Bread (*See last Chapter Six for discussion of both*)

1 and a-half cup yogurt-soymilk mixture (half nonfat plain yogurt and half plain unsweetened soymilk)

Sliced carrot sticks, raw

Peanut butter is cold and stiff from being in the refrigerator, which makes it a little hard to spread evenly. Normally, I don't worry about it and spread it on pretty thick. When I'm peaking, however, I take time to put a dollop in the microwave for about 30 seconds. This allows me to spread the peanut butter more evenly. That saves a few calories, and doesn't seem to make any difference in eating satisfaction—exactly what I'm trying to achieve. I also have a little more soymilk (about 1 cup) and a little less yogurt (about a half cup), another painless calorie-saving tradeoff.

Mid-Afternoon Snack

1 Tiger's Milk Nutrition Bar (comes in protein or peanut butter; I prefer the protein)

1 and a-half cup plain unsweetened soymilk

I cut back to 1 cup soymilk and add a little water; a reduction of about 40 calories—and barely noticeable.

Dinner

Large mixed green salad (prepared by Carol)
   Romaine lettuce, chopped
   Celery, chopped
   Mushrooms, sliced
   Cucumber, sliced
   Grape tomatoes
   Green bell pepper, diced
   Radishes, sliced
   Avocado, about one heaping tablespoon
   Olive oil, 1 teaspoon
   Balsamic vinegar, two teaspoons
2 poached eggs or broiled fish or skinless chicken breast
2 Slices Sprouted Grain Bread w/ Benecol Light Spread
Baked sweet potato, several slices
I drop one slice of bread, 80 calories. (The eggs, broiled fish,

and skinless chicken breast are interchangeable and have about the same number of calories.)

Bedtime Snack

One slice Sprouted Grain Bread topped with thinly spread almond butter, Benecol, and a little honey

This is delicious and I don't change it. Ignore those who tell you not to eat anything after a certain hour in the evening. Telling yourself you can't have something only makes you want it, even if you wouldn't miss it otherwise. Plan your bedtime snack. Look forward to it. Enjoy it. (Don't skip it.) Total calories over the course of the day are what counts.

These portions, of course, are mine. You may need more or less, depending on your bodyweight, muscle mass, and activity level. Again, the take-home message is to make small changes that your fat cells will notice, but you won't. And do it consistently.

And don't forget: Only put on the table what you plan to eat. Clear everything else away before you start eating. (See Chapter Three)

* * * *

This chapter explained that healthy eating and dieting to achieve peak condition are essentially one and the same; the only difference is more consistency and precision when peaking or striving to become leaner for any reason. I recommended that you buy a body composition monitor and explained how it can help track your progress. The key is to understand how your monitor works and accept that all methods are informed estimates; weigh yourself under the same circumstances each time and focus on tracking change in response to diet and exercise. We went over my body composition readings and discussed what I normally eat and how I modify my meals to create a small calorie deficit and start my body fat on a downward path. It's very important to take your time and not rush the process.

Now let's talk about training to look and feel your best. I'll explain my philosophy on training and peaking, and tell you how I trained to peak at 70. (It's not fundamentally different than how I've been training for decades.) We'll also have a few words on injuries.

Gym lore holds that the best way to get into top shape is to train longer and lighter. In my experience, that's wrong.

Chapter Eight

Training for the Peak

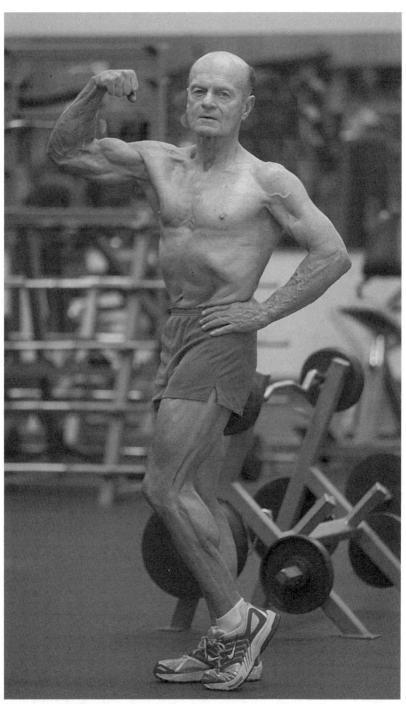

At Liberty Gym in Albuquerque, NM. *Photo by Laszlo Bencze*

Training Philosophy

As in the case of diet, training to achieve peak condition (for any important event or occasion) is different only in intensity and focus. I'll begin with my general philosophy on training.

I started exercising when I was about 13—and never stopped. I look on training as a lifetime pursuit. I believe your body tends to mirror your lifestyle. That's nature's way. The body seems to sense that an active person needs to be lean and muscular, and conversely, that a sedentary person does not.

I take a long-term approach to exercise, an approach designed to keep me training—and improving—year after year.

Weight training has always been my first love. But I recognize that one cannot be totally fit without aerobic exercise. Therefore, I follow a balanced exercise program: strength and endurance. A dual approach, weights and aerobics, is not only necessary for total fitness; it's also the best way to achieve peak condition.

Enjoyment, believe it or not, is the key ingredient in any really successful exercise plan. That doesn't mean the program must be easy. To the contrary, productive exercise is often brutally hard. What it does mean is that the regimen must be satisfying.

In my view, exercise satisfaction comes mainly from two things: variety, and setting and achieving goals. Both the body and the mind respond best to a varied exercise approach. Variation keeps your body responding and is essential to long-term progress.

Goals, realistic goals, are equally important, because they keep you motivated. Nothing is more satisfying than to set an exercise goal or target, work hard, and then achieve that goal. But a goal achieved is a goal lost, so you must continually challenge yourself with new goals, workout to workout, and long term.

Finally, I don't have all day to spend in the gym. I have a life outside the gym, and I know my readers do as well. Fortunately, that's never been a problem, because in my experience best results come from short, hard, and infrequent training—weights and aerobics.

None of this changes when training to achieve top condition. A few things need to be emphasized, however.

Peaking

In Chapter Five, paraphrasing Arthur Jones, I said that more exercise is rarely the answer for a dedicated trainer. That's still true when training for peak condition.

Gym lore holds that the best way to get into top shape is to train longer and lighter—to burn off fat and become more defined. In my experience, that's wrong. Peak condition for a bodybuilder (or anyone striving to look their best) means leaner and stronger, which go hand in hand.

Training lighter and longer (less resistance and more sets and reps) generally means using fewer muscle fibers. And muscle fibers that aren't being used are likely to be lost—use it or lose it. Diet and aerobics are the best way to lose fat; and hard, brief weight training is the best way to build and retain muscle. (Muscle mass drives metabolism, so weight training also aids fat loss.)

Overload remains a prime requisite (weights and aerobics). Simply stated, you must continually strive to improve on your past performance. Do that, gradually and progressively, and you will become stronger and fitter, and look better.

Progressive overload remains the key when peaking, because strength loss signals muscle loss. You must continue to challenge your body to become stronger and fitter. That doesn't mean you must make progress every workout, of course. It's okay to repeat or even back off occasionally. When you hit a sticking point, it's often best to pull back and build up again.

If you find yourself getting weaker, it's almost always time to go back to the drawing board. You are probably overtraining—too much stress and not enough rest—or undereating.

When peaking, continue to focus on overload and rest. Strive to not only look your best, but also to become stronger and fitter. As noted earlier, looks and performance can and should go hand in hand.

My Training Routine

Like the meals in the last chapter, this routine is not magic; it is, however, a fundamentally sound and complete training plan. It's the routine that evolved as I was getting back into regular training after my hip replacement. It's different than anything I've written about before, and a good basic routine for peaking— or anytime really. It's a routine that a broad spectrum of people, serious trainers of any age, can use or draw ideas from. It also gives me an opportunity to tell about some new things I've tried recently—and how I've adjusted to my new hip and some other common problems.

Let's start with the daily breakdown. Notice the simplicity and balance: three workouts, equal emphasis on strength and aerobics, and three or four days of active rest.

Sunday	Whole body weights
Monday	Walk
Tuesday	Walk
Wednesday	Upper body strength, lower body aerobics
Thursday	Walk
Friday	Walk (or rest)
Saturday	Whole body aerobics

This scheme may not look like much, but it's more sophisticated than it seems at first glance. One-and-a-half weight workouts would please Arthur Jones. Bill Bowerman would probably like one-and-a-half aerobic workouts—and the walking (hard/easy). And George Sheehan would appreciate the overall stress-to-rest ratio.

Each workout is different; there's plenty of variety to challenge the body and mind. The Sunday weight session is probably the most traditional, and a good place to start looking at the details.

Whole-Body Weights

General Warm-up (elbows, shoulders, knees, hips, lower back)
Leg Extension
Leg Curl
Seated or Standing Calf Raise (alternate week to week)
Machine Pullover (optional)
Lat Pulldown (grip optional)
One-Arm Dumbbell Row
Dumbbell Bench Press
Incline Barbell Press
Standing Pulley Fly
Upright Dumbbell Row
Dumbbell Shrug
Barbell or Dumbbell Curl
Slant-Board Hip Curl (option Reverse Crunch)
Kneeling Side-to-Side Rope Pulldown (option One-Arm DB Sidebend)
General Cooldown (same as warm-up)

The general warm-up (and cooldown) is what the name implies: a simple and logical warm-up of the whole body. I flex and extend all my joints about ten times to loosen up and get the blood flowing—without weights. This little routine also helps me get in the mood to train and wind down at the end of the workout. I bend and extend my elbows, shrug my shoulders, swing my arms (like swimming), curl my legs and lift my knees (see photo), stretch my back and hamstrings, and squat. It only takes a few minutes, but it's important; it prepares your mind and body to train. I do it before and after every workout. (I often do it in the morning after I shave to help get my day off to a good start.)

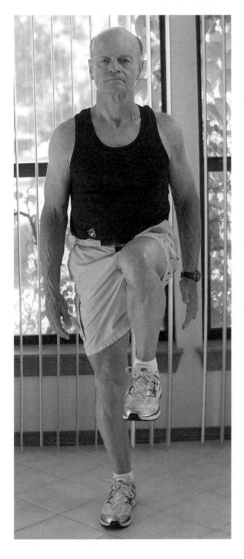

This is the knee lift I do as part of my general warm-up. I do a standing leg curl and then the knee lift, to loosen my knees and hips. The other movements are just as straightforward. Move to loosen-up all your joints and get your blood flowing. There's no special way to do it. Use your imagination, but don't do anything that hurts.
Photo by Laszlo Bencze

If you need help with these or the other exercises, you'll find books on the performance of standard lifting movements on our website (www.cbass.com) or in most bookstores. Another alternative is to hire a personal trainer to help you get started.

That brings us to the obvious question. Where are the cornerstone movements in my previous weight workouts: the squat and

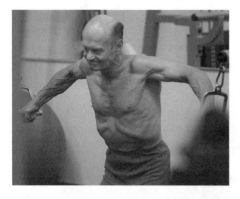

This is the Standing Pulley Fly; it works the outer and lower part of the chest. If you don't have access to a cross-over pulley, you can substitute lying dumbbell flies, or parallel-bar dips, or just skip it. The flat and incline bench press with barbell or dumbbell work the chest adequately. *Photo by Laszlo Bencze*

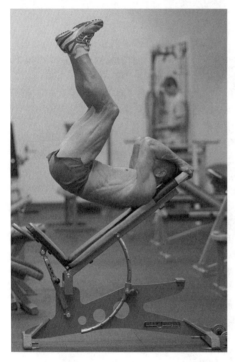

The Slant-Board Hip Curl works the lower abdominal muscles. The top position is shown here; lower your hips to the bench and curl back up—you'll feel it in the lower part of your torso. You can substitute hanging knee raises, or the reverse crunch, where you raise the hips rather than the shoulders; lie on your back with your feet flat on the floor, and lift or curl your hips using your abdominal muscles. *Photo by Laszlo Bencze*

deadlift? It's not what you think. I don't believe my hip would keep me from doing these movements. My power-lifter friend Rickey Dale Crain, who's about my size, worked up to 505 pounds in the squat during the first year after having his hip replaced; it makes his doctor a little nervous, but he's now aiming for 600. I'm not saying that's necessarily a good idea, but it suggests what's possible.

The problem is "moderate-to-mild" osteoarthritis in my lower back. I pinched some nerves in my spine bending awkwardly while rehabbing my hip—and now compression of my lower

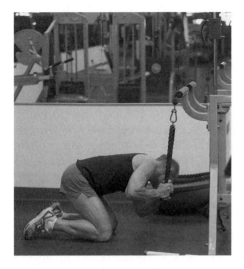

The Kneeling Side-to-Side Rope Pulldown works the muscles on the sides of your waist. Pulldown to one side of your head and then the other; control the weight throughout the motion, up and down. You'll feel it in the muscles on both sides. The Dumbbell Sidebend is a substitute. *Photo by Laszlo Bencze*

back makes my feet numb. My neurologist *suggested* that I avoid movements that compress my lower back. (I've heard from many trainers who have the same problem. Many of them can do leg presses if they are careful.)

Happily, I have found a way to work my lower back, hips, and hamstrings quite effectively without doing squats or deadlifts. I'll tell you how when we get to the Wednesday and Saturday workouts. (I also do leg presses as part of my Sunday workout about twice a month—the same frequency as I did squats previously.)

In Chapter 5, I hinted at the other major change in this routine. I never thought I would enjoy slow lifting, but that's what has happened. It's not super slow by any means, but I am doing a form of slow lifting.

I read what Ell Darden said about slow reps in his new book, and tried it when I strained my elbow doing the incline barbell press. To my surprise, the slow reps made my shoulders and triceps sore; obviously something new and different was happening. I liked the response and tried it on the other exercises in this workout.

To make a long story short, I now do slow reps in this workout every other week: one week regular reps and slow the next. I like the variety and believe it may improve my results. I know my elbow and other joints like the slow reps. I plan to keep lifting slow every other week as long as my body keeps responding to the variation.

I don't time rep speed, however; that would be a drag and I don't believe it's necessary. As noted earlier, Arthur Jones did not recommend timing reps. On the "regular" week, I do the exercises like I've always done them, at the speed that feels best to me; I control the weight up and down, but make no effort to slow rep speed. On the "slow" week, I make a special effort to start each rep under control, no jerking, and not increase the speed as the movement continues—just as Jones recommended.

As Darden relates in his book, this translates into about two seconds up and four seconds down. The actual time probably varies from exercise to exercise. I don't know precisely how much slower my slow reps are, but I can definitely feel the difference. My plan is to keep changing rep speed from week to week as long I enjoy it and the muscle response is good. As I said earlier, variety challenges the body and mind. Change is good.

I do one or two warm-up sets (usually 4-8 reps) with moderate weight, and one hard work set. The work-set reps are generally from 6 to 15. Reps and poundages in the "slow" week are about 15% lower, because slow reps take longer and are more fatiguing than regular reps.

As indicated early on in this chapter, I increase reps or weight whenever I can. When necessary, however, I don't hesitate to repeat what I did the last workout or back off when I get ahead of myself. I check my training diary before every workout and write down what I did last time; this gives me a target for every exercise. (More about use of the training diary later in this chapter)

Strictly speaking, I am not using periodization (cycles of programmed change). But I am in a sense, because (as noted) I back off in reps or weight when I get ahead of myself or encountering a sticking point. I try never to fail. I know when I can't do another rep in good form, and stop. If I'm not able to increase for several workouts in a row, I usually reduce the resistance and start up again. In fact, as I write this I've just reduced poundages across the board to begin a steady increase in resistance leading into to a full week of photos for this book.

You might call what I'm doing *free style periodization*. I always keep in mind Bill Pearl's sage advice to save a little for next time. If I can't go up in resistance, I retreat in preparation for another slow build-up. Planning for success almost always works. It sure beats repeated failure—which is a major motivation killer.

Let's move on to the Wednesday workout, which is something new, for me anyway.

Upper-Body Strength, Lower-Body Aerobics

General Warm-up (same as before)
Glute-Ham Raise (lower body, but works well here, with Lifecycle)

Seated Lat Pull
Seated Chest Press
Seated Shoulder Press
Side-to-Side Crunch
Lifecycle
General Cooldown

This workout is just what the name says. On Wednesday, I train the upper body for strength and the lower body for aerobic fitness. I train the upper body twice in the same week (Sunday and Wednesday), because the smaller muscles of the upper body recover from strength training faster than the large muscles of the lower body. The upper body can benefit from more volume and variety; not a lot more, however. So be careful.

As the authors of *Younger Next Year* observed (in Chapter 4), recovery from endurance training generally occurs overnight. That's true for walking or jogging, but this is high-intensity aerobics. In my experience, recovery from high-intensity aerobics takes longer. The aerobic training here and on Saturday includes intervals; it's hard. I do it one-and-a-half times a week, just like the strength training. (Endurance athletes typically restrict interval training to once or, at most, twice a week.)

This combination workout may be too much for some people. If you don't feel recovered from the weekend workouts, you can go easy on this workout or even skip it entirely—and walk. As Bill Bowerman taught, it's better to do too little than too much.

The Glute Ham Developer

The Glute-Ham Raise, the first exercise after the general warm-up, is the first of two exercises I use to replace the squat and deadlift. I referred to this movement in Chapter 2; it is one of the exercises I used before my hip replacement and planned to resume using afterward. It's performed on a relatively inexpensive apparatus called the "Glute Ham Developer," which we purchased from Bigger Faster Stronger (BFS), a company located in Salt Lake City, Utah (www.biggerfasterstronger.com). You'll find it or a similar unit in many commercial gyms. Those that don't have access to this equipment can do something similar by lying face down over the end of a flat bench, and have a friend hold your feet down. (Be careful.)

The BFS booklet says the Glute Ham Developer makes possible "the ONLY exercise that maximally develops the gluteus maximus and hamstring muscles." That may be a bit of a stretch, but it does provide the most concentrated stress on the glutes (butt) and hamstrings I have ever experienced.

These photos show how the Glut-Ham Raise is done: Adjust the foot plate so your hips extend slightly beyond the curved pad, and lower your upper body about half way, bending at the hips (keep your back straight); pull yourself up by extending your hips, and then flexing

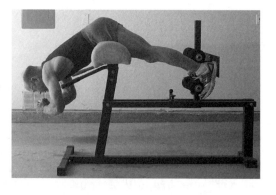

your hamstrings (like a leg curl); contract your glutes (butt) hard at the top. Trust me; you'll know when you get it right; you'll feel an intense contraction in your glutes, and then in your leg biceps. Be sure to fully extend your body (straighten your knees) on each rep to get a full range motion.

Do a few reps to warm-up, and then do one work set; start with about 10 controlled reps (whatever you can do comfortably) and work up to 40-50 controlled reps; when you can do more than 50 reps, hold a weight plate in front of your chest or face (not behind your neck). Focus on bodyweight reps with this exercise, because we'll add weight on Saturday when doing the Back Raise.

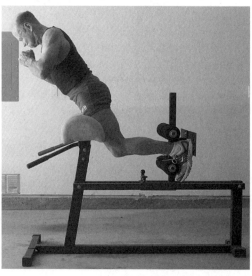

Photos by Laszlo Bencze

I do the next three exercises on Keiser compressor-resistance machines, but they are basic movements; any standard machine or free weights will work. I do one or two warm-up sets with light to medium resistance, and one work set of 8 to 12 reps; I gradually increase the resistance as I get stronger. As in the Sunday workout, I do regular speed reps one week and slow reps the next.

120

The following photos show me doing the seated row, chest press, and shoulder press on Keiser machines. Again, they are basic movements which can be done on other machines or with barbells and dumbbells.

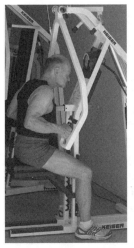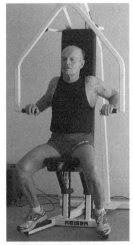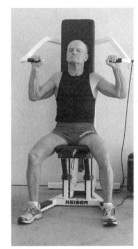

Photos by Laszlo Bencze

The final strength exercise is the side-to-side crunch, which is simply a three-way crunch with your knees bent and your feet flat on the floor. If you can do more than 50 total reps, hold a weight plate behind your neck (use a pad for comfort and to support your neck). Curl up at three angles: center, right, center, left and so on. In other words, come straight up on the first rep, to the right on the next rep, center again, and then left. The idea is to work the side muscles (the external obliques) as well as the muscles in the front (the rectus abdominis). You don't have to twist very far; just enough to feel the tension on the sides. Done properly, the movement will work the front and both sides of your waist very effectively. You'll like how it feels. Remember: Don't pull on your neck. Use the weight plate and pad to keep your neck straight (like a splint).

I use less resistance and more reps on Wednesday, and then do the regular crunch (coming straight up) on Saturday with more weight and fewer reps. I generally use about 10 pounds on Wednesday and do 50 or 60 reps. On Saturday, I double the weight and do 30 or 40 reps. There's no magic number; just do enough reps to fully tire the waist muscles. Using more resistance on Saturday makes it more interesting and provides a different stress. Again, your muscles (and your mind) thrive on variety. Do full-range reps and contract your abs hard on every rep.

Lifecycle

Now we come to the lower-body aerobics in the Wednesday workout—the hardest and most challenging part. I have a bit of a love-hate relationship with the Lifecycle. I hate to get on, but love how spent and satisfied I feel at the end—all in about 20 minutes. Actually, it's a real deal. It's what Chris and Harry call the second and third gears our ancient ancestors used for hunting and "escape or capture" situations—and you don't have to kill anything or anybody. You do have to be careful, however, especially if you're not in pretty good shape. Be sure to talk to your doctor if you have any health concerns.

The simplest way to use the Lifecycle, or any computerized stationary bicycle, is to follow one of the programmed workouts. The hill program is a favorite on most exercise bikes; I've used it many times and like it.

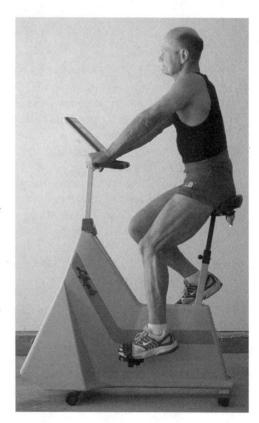

Any program with intervals is fine. I prefer the manual setting, however, because it gives me second-by-second flexibility to shape my own workout and gradually ratchet up intensity—or pull back if necessary. The workout that follows is one of my favorites; it's based on a load-level range of 1-12, with 1 being the easiest and 12 the hardest. *Photo by Laszlo Bencze*

```
5-minute warm-up at level 1
30 seconds. . . . . . . . . . . . . .2
30s. . . . . . . . . . . . . . . . . .3
30s. . . . . . . . . . . . . . . . . .4
30s. . . . . . . . . . . . . . . . . .5
30s. . . . . . . . . . . . . . . . . .6
30s. . . . . . . . . . . . . . . . . .7
2 min. . . . . . . . . . . . . . . .1
1 min. . . . . . . . . . . . . . . .7
90s. . . . . . . . . . . . . . . . . .1
30s. . . . . . . . . . . . . . . . . .8
90s. . . . . . . . . . . . . . . . . .1
30s. . . . . . . . . . . . . . . . . .9
5-min cooldown. . . . . . . . . .1
```

Total = 20 minutes

This format can be easily altered to make it harder or easier. Here are some examples: The stairs after the 5-minute warm-up can be made longer or shorter; for example, you can cut the length of the steps to 20 seconds or increase them to 45 seconds or one minute. You can add another step at level 8, or drop the step at level 6. You can adjust any of the intervals after the steps by shortening or lengthening the rest or work periods; you can, of course, raise or lower the load level. You have complete control to create your own workout plan. And you can always change the plan anytime during the workout.

I use all of these options, but I do it gradually, rarely changing more than one or two variables at a time. My first adjustment is usually to add or subtract a step; after that, I usually increase (or decrease) the load level on one or more of the 30s intervals in the last half of the workout, or add another 30s interval at a higher level.

I sit down with my training diary and plan what I'm going to do before each workout, but always reserve (and often exercise) the option to make changes on the fly during the workout. Use your options well; make each workout a challenging—and positive—experience. *Photo by Laszlo Bencze*

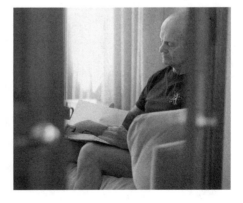

Like diet changes, it's best to make small, manageable changes; don't bite off more than you can chew. Make each workout *slightly* harder (or easier); be careful not to overreach and stall your progress. Always fine-tune for success.

If you are still harboring the notion that this doesn't seem like much of a workout, perish the thought. Match the intensity level to your strength and fitness level, and you'll be breathing hard on the last step and during every 30s work period (that's why they're called work periods). Your quads will be on fire during the last work interval.

You'll be glad to begin the 5-minute cooldown; actually you'll want to skip the cooldown and lie down. But don't do it! The cooldown keeps the blood from pooling in your legs; it helps to gradually return your heart and body to normal. Don't skip the cooldown.

Okay, you say, but why only 20 minutes? Isn't this supposed to be the aerobic part of the workout? Keep in mind that we're not training for the Tour de France. This is a balanced workout, strength and endurance. Too much endurance training can use up precious recovery capacity and break down muscle tissue. My objective, and probably yours, is to get the fat-burning and fitness benefits of aerobic exercise—without detracting from the strength portion of the routine. Relatively short and infrequent interval workouts, like this one, are the best way to do that.

(Don't forget to talk to your doctor if you have any health problems. If you are new to exercise, start slowly and give your body plenty of time to adjust.)

Now, let's move on to the Saturday workout.

Whole-Body Aerobics

General Warm-up (same as before)
Back Raise with added weight
Crunch
Saxon Sidebend
Schwinn Airdyne
General Cooldown

(The Back Raise and the ab exercises are, of course, not aerobic. I include them in my Saturday workout simply because it's convenient and works well.)

The Back Raise is done on the same apparatus as the Glute-Ham Raise in the Wednesday workout. The difference is that the foot plate is a little farther back so that your hips are squarely on the curved pad. Again, lower the upper body about half way and come back up, this time using *only* your lower back and hips.

(The hamstrings work only as stabilizers and are not flexed; the knees remain straight.)

The BFS booklet says to go all the way down and flex (round) the back—but I don't. I only go down about half way and keep my back straight or slightly arched, just as I would in the squat or deadlift. (Previous photo shows bottom position) My sports medicine specialist, Dr. Wilson, told me not to round my lower back; he says it might pinch or inflame the nerves coming out of my arthritic spine. If your back is okay, you can probably go all the way down, rounding your back somewhat. Just be careful.

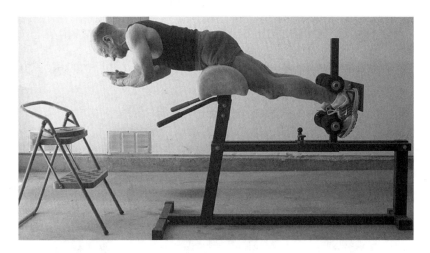

Either way, keep your legs straight. Bending the knees puts the stress on the hamstrings; you don't want that. This movement is for your low back and hips, not your leg biceps. Come up until your body is straight, parallel to the floor; pause briefly at the top of each rep and tense or squeeze your butt. Don't hyperextend your back. (Photo shows proper position; look carefully and you'll see the weight plates, in my hands and on the stool.)

This is a terrific exercise. Do it in a controlled manner (don't jerk) and you'll feel a strong contraction in your lower back and hips. Allow some time to get used to the movement, and then add weight as necessary. Because of the leverage factor, you won't need much weight; hold the weight under your nose, as shown in the photo.

I do three warm-up sets of about 10 reps, the first without weight and the second and third holding a weight plate (5 kilos and then 10 kilos, or 11 and 22 pounds), and then a work set of 10-20 reps with 15 kilos (33 pounds). When I can do 20 controlled reps, I add 1.25-2.5 kilos (roughly 2.5-5 pounds), drop back to 10 reps and work up again. You'll need more or less weight, depending on your size and strength. Remember to increase the resistance as you become stronger.

As you'll remember, I do this exercise as a substitute for the squat and deadlift, because compression on my spine causes numbness in my feet. I know that many people have the same problem. (If your back is healthy and you prefer, you can substitute squats and deadlifts for the Back Raise and the Glute-Ham Raise, respectively. I suggest that this be done at the beginning of the Sunday weight workout, doing the squat one week and the deadlift the next. You can drop the leg extension and leg curl if you like. Only experienced lifters should consider this option. Others can substitute the leg press.)

Moving on to the crunch, I use about 20 pounds behind my neck, and curl straight up (no side-to-side motion). I do 40-50 reps, or until my abs are tired. Again, knees bent and feet flat on the floor.

Saxon Sidebends

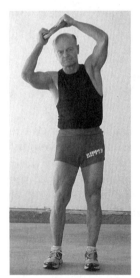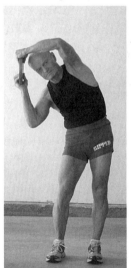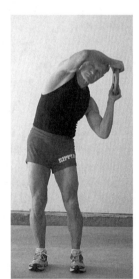

Photos by Laszlo Bencze

The Saxon sidebend is a sidebend holding a weight plate or dumbbell overhead. (See photos) Because of the leverage factor, you don't need much weight. I warm-up without weight, and then do about 10 reps with a 5-kilo plate and about 25 with 10 kilos. Do controlled reps and bend directly to the side (right and left) as far as you can; keep your legs straight, don't bend your knees. Take your time getting used to the movement—don't hurt yourself. It works the muscles on both sides of the waist, your obliques. (No, it won't overdevelop your waist.) Bend your arms and hold the weight just above the head; let the weight move from side to side in a natural manner. The idea is to firm your sides, not work the arms.

Schwinn Airdyne

Readers of my earlier books are familiar with the Schwinn Airdyne, a stationary bike that works the whole body. (See Photo below) I am frequently asked whether it is still my favorite aerobic exercise device. It is, yes, absolutely, because it suits the needs of almost everyone. (Carol and I are on our third Airdyne.) The distinguishing feature is the push-pull arm action. Wind vanes in the wheel allow you to make your own resistance; like riding a bike outdoors, the faster you pedal, push and pull, the harder it is. Time and resistance (load level) are tracked on the digital performance monitor.

You'll find the Airdyne in many fitness centers, and you can buy one for a very reasonable price at most fitness equipment stores. (You can read more about the Airdyne in my book *Lean For Life*, or check out the latest models on Google. I've told you all you really need to know.)

The workout is similar to what we did on the Lifecycle. The difference is that arms and legs are worked together and separately. That's an important feature, because the benefit of aerobic exercise occurs mainly in the muscles being used; for the most part, the rest of the body just goes along for the ride. (The heart, lungs, and circulatory system also benefit, of course.) The Airdyne builds strength, aerobic fitness, and fat-burning capacity in the whole body.

Here's one of my favorite workout plans. Unless otherwise indicated, all segments are arms and legs.

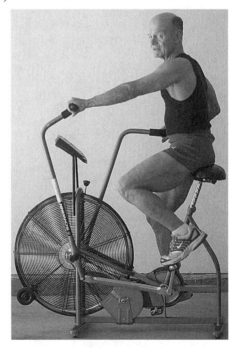

Photo by Laszlo Bencze

127

Level 1 on the monitor is very easy and 10 is very hard. (I don't know how high the monitor will register; I've only seen one person register 10, and that was a short sprint.)

5 Minutes gradual warm-up at Load Level 1-3
30 seconds 3.5
30s 4.0
30s 4.5
30s 5.0
30s 5.5
30s 6.0
1:30 min. 1.5
30s 4.0
30s 5.0
30s 6.0
1:30 min. 1.5
30s . . . . .3.0 (Arms Only)
30s . . . . .4.5 (Legs Only)
30s . . . . .6.0 (Arms & Legs)
2 min 1.5
1 min 6.0
5 min cooldown 1.0
Total = 22 minutes

Everything I said about the Lifecycle workout applies here as well. Feel free to alter the format. Whether you use my plan

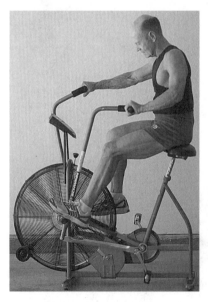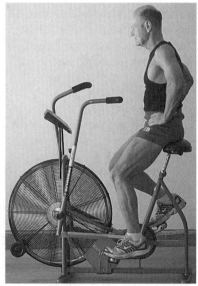

Photos by Laszlo Bencze

128

or design your own, start at a comfortable pace and increase intensity slowly and gradually as your fitness improves—and don't hesitate to reduce the load level if you hit a sticking point or overreach and get ahead of yourself. I frequently back off when the going gets tough, and then work up again. This works much better than trying to push past your limit and failing repeatedly. A cyclical up-and-down training plan will get you a lot farther down the road in the long run—and you'll enjoy it more.

I really like the Arms Only and Legs Only segments. They break up the workout and make it more interesting—and add a different and challenging strength aspect. Don't overdo arms or legs only, however, because it can interrupt your rhythm and ruin the workout; you might not be able to complete the workout. I find that one bout of arms only and one of legs only is enough; remember that the main advantage of the Airdyne is that it works the whole body at one time. Whatever you do, plan your workouts for success, and try never to fail.

Now, let's talk about walking on off days.

Walking

Don't skip the walking part of the overall training plan. Walking burns some extra calories and fat, but that's only part of the story, and not even the most important part. Remember what Dr. Harry Lodge said about light aerobic exercise (up to 65% of VO2max) in *Younger Next Year*? Walking and foraging, he said, is "the metabolic zone where your body and brain heal and grow." He called it "a wonderful pace."

I usually walk about 30-40 minutes on the days when I don't work out, and up to an hour when I'm peaking for photos. Harry is absolutely right. Walking helps me recover faster, and makes me feel good and think better. I always make time for my walks. (Carol is also an avid walker and hiker.)

About Injuries

My earlier books included little or nothing about injuries, for the simple reason that my training has been essentially injury free; a few aches and pains that come with an active lifestyle, but not much more. In light of recent developments, discussed in Chapter 2, it seems appropriate to delve into the subject now. I'll warn you that I still don't have a lot to offer. What follows will seem like simple common sense, because that's what it is. I'm not a doctor or a physical therapist, just a guy who has been training successfully for a very long time.

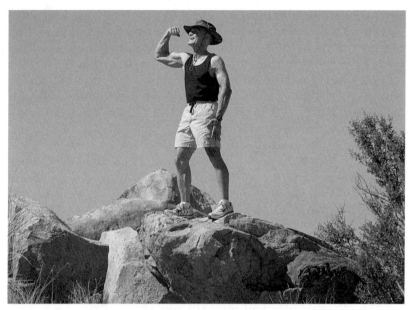

Walking just makes you feel good. *Photo by Laszlo Bencze*

What I have said in the past still goes: *If it hurts don't do it.* That's my guiding principle. And I take my own advice most of the time. (Like anyone else, I get carried away at times—and usually pay the price.) Attempting to train through pain is almost always a bad idea. You'll do far better in the long run if you take a break and let even a minor injury heal. My experience is that you can find a way to train around most injuries; and that's what I've done. (Switching to the Glute Ham Developer, before and after my hip replacement, is an example.) Complete inactivity is rarely necessary or wise.

I try to move an injured area *under the pain threshold* whenever possible. Motion without pain promotes circulation and speeds healing. I do it in the morning after I shave or while I'm walking; something as simple as bending a sore elbow back and forth, moving a gimpy shoulder, or flexing and extending a banged-up knee can help a lot to speed healing. Motion that feels good usually is.

In later years, I've tried icing hot (sore) spots, minor pulls, or strains. I apply ice as soon as possible after a workout, for 10-15 minutes, using "hi tech" bags of frozen peas or other small veggies from our freezer. It's a nuisance, but does seem to help control inflammation and promote healing. (For serious injuries, go to the emergency room or call your doctor for advice.).

I try to avoid non-steroidal anti-inflammatory drugs (NSAIDs), such as Advil and Aleve, because they cause constipation and can raise blood pressure; some studies suggest that they may even be bad for the heart. I don't believe anyone knows for sure about the more serious side-effects, but it's probably better to be safe than sorry. I have used Advil and Aleve for minor aches and pains on a temporary basis (they work), and I would again.

If your injury doesn't heal after a reasonable time using the conservative methods we've discussed, it's probably time to see an orthopedist or sports medicine specialist for a proper diagnosis and appropriate treatment. For more serious injuries, of course, seek immediate help.

* * * *

Here we talked about training, day-to-day and when peaking. As in the case of diet, the two are different only in intensity and focus. More is usually not better, even when peaking. We highlighted progressive overload and rest, which take on special importance when peaking. I described and explained my own training program, not because I believe you should follow it to the letter, but to give you ideas to consider for your own training. Finally, we discussed dealing with minor injuries.

Now, let's talk about motivation and change. No program can succeed unless you are motivated to begin, stick with it, and change when necessary.

"Periods of struggling to overcome challenges are what people find to be the most enjoyable times of their lives."

Mihaly Csikszentmihalyi,
PhD

"I do not believe that you should devote overly much effort to correcting your weaknesses. Rather, I believe that the highest success in living and the deepest emotional satisfaction comes from building and using your signature strengths."

Martin E. P. Seligman, PhD

"Fitness is a journey, not a destination. And it starts with the first step."

Cooper Clinic

Chapter Nine

Motivation and Change

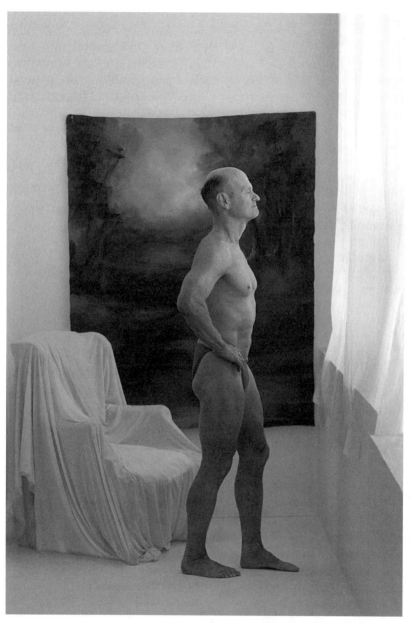

Photo by Laszlo Bencze

Plan for Success

Change is hard. The only program, diet or exercise, that will work is one you are willing and able to stick with until it's time to change again.

People get fired up about losing fat and becoming fit and healthy. They charge in with arms and legs flailing—and promptly fall on their face. It's like starting a marathon at top speed. No one can maintain such a pace. Rushing the process leads to discouragement and failure. It's why most fitness plans are abandoned in weeks or, at most, months.

Forget "No pain, no gain." Suffering is not required or even desirable. Pain and suffering are a prescription for failure.

Fitness is not a destination. It's a continuing process, a wonderful journey of discovery that begins with the first step and, ideally, never ends.

Start slowly, at a pace you know you can maintain. Experience success early on and then build on your success.

Plan for success. Start with motivation.

Motivation is the sine qua non of success. It's essential. Without motivation you are dead in the water. The key to sustained motivation is enjoyment—or flow.

Flow Revisited

It is just common sense: If you enjoy an activity, you're likely to stick with it. If you don't enjoy something, you'll probably decide it's not worth the effort and stop doing it.

What makes an activity like training enjoyable? (Hint, it's not turning it into a cake walk.)

I've written before about the importance of *flow*, a term coined by psychologist Mihaly Csikszentmihalyi, PhD, but it's worth reviewing here; for those learning about it for the first time, it's fundamental to success in any ongoing pursuit.

In his landmark book *Flow: The Psychology of Optimal Experience*, (Harper & Row, 1990), Csikszentmihalyi (Dr. C to me) related a powerful truth known since the days of Aristotle: "Periods of struggling to overcome challenges are what people find to be the most enjoyable times of their lives."

Flow is the term he uses to describe those times when people report feelings of enjoyment, concentration, and deep involvement, or a genuinely enjoyable state of consciousness. Paraphrasing Dr. C, here's the blueprint followed by people who experience flow: They set appropriate goals, closely monitor feedback, and when they reach their goal, they up the ante, setting increasingly complex challenges for themselves.

Applied to training, that means essentially three things: Set reasonable but challenging goals, monitor progress, and (this is important) never forget that a goal achieved is a goal lost. You must keep setting meaningful new goals.

I believe that three-pronged formula explains why I'm still going strong after more than 55 years of high-level training. My athletic and fitness career is built on finding and pursuing activities I find enjoyable and challenging. With that as my cornerstone, by intuition and good fortune in my early years and by design in recent years, I've gone from success to success.

Let's talk about the short term—the next workout—and then the long term.

On a short-term basis, I go into each workout with a plan. I sit down with my training diary and set specific goals for each exercise. I take the diary to the gym and record what I do—and set goals for next time. That's the Flow formula in microcosm, isn't it? Set goal, record feedback, and set new goal.

That doesn't mean I try to improve in every exercise every workout. I don't; that would be unrealistic. Every workout should be a positive experience; one that makes you want to return to the gym—again and again.

When necessary, I don't hesitate to repeat what I did last time

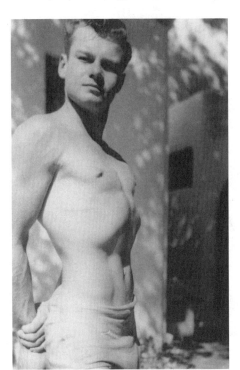

or even back off a little. I strive for as much positive feedback as possible. Failure, especially repeated failure, kills motivation; I try to avoid it. I always train with an eye to the next workout. Following Bill Pearl's sage advice, I almost always "save a little for next time."

I see the gym as an inviting place, and I want to keep it that way.

By age 15, the results of my training were showing clearly in this photo taken by my dad.

On a long-term basis, I look for areas in which I can excel, or at least improve. Like most beginners, my body responded well to training; my sessions with my dad's weights when I was in the fifth and sixth grades were productive and rewarding. Looking back now, I realize that they were life-changing; they established a pattern of success that has served me well ever since.

Psychologist Martin E. P. Seligman, PhD, a student of Dr. C's and the leading spokesman for the new movement of Positive Psychology, which focuses on mental health rather than mental illness, wrote in *Authentic Happiness* (Free Press, 2002): "I do not believe that you should devote overly much effort to correcting your weaknesses. Rather, I believe that the highest success in living and the deepest emotional satisfaction comes from building and using your signature strengths."

I knew early on that I liked lifting weights to develop muscle and get stronger. I was built for lifting and activities requiring strength; I wasn't cut out to run marathons. I found what I did well and stuck with it. Dr. Seligman, I'm sure, would agree that finding a sport you enjoy is a key to long-term success. That doesn't mean you have to be a champion; it simply means you'll do better in an activity that you find rewarding and satisfying.

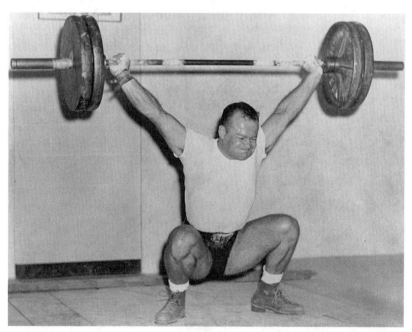

It didn't take me long to master the squat-style snatch, one of the three Olympic lifts contested at that time; here I'm shown snatching 225 pounds in a statewide competition.

Satisfaction, for most people, comes from making progress, being successful in a continuing competition with yourself.

Dr. C, you'll remember, found that successful people, those that experience *flow,* set increasingly complex challenges for themselves. That's what I have done.

Capitalizing on the gains made in my bedroom, I trained for and won the New Mexico State High School Pentathlon championship, a five-event strength and fitness competition held in conjunction with the state track and field championship. A recap of the year in high school sports by our local newspaper included the sub-title: "Bass is strongest." We still have the clipping.

Using that success as a steppingstone, I moved on to Olympic weightlifting. Over roughly two decades, I won at the city, state, and regional level, and placed high in national competition.

When I topped out as an Olympic lifter in my mid-30s, I moved on to physique competition, where there was plenty of room for improvement. After several years of bodybuilding training, I entered local competition and eventually won the "Most Muscular Man" award in open statewide competition.

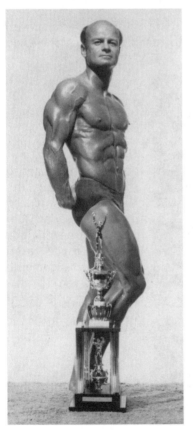

Encouraged by that success, I moved on to national age-group competition, where I won my class in both the Past-40 Mr. America and the Past-40 Mr. USA. In the latter competition, I again won the overall "Most Muscular Man" award.

The 1980 Past-40 Mr. America, where I placed second as a middleweight, was my last venture into bodybuilding competition, but I have never stopped trying to improve my physique, as shown by the current photos appearing throughout this book.

Here I am in 1978, winning my class at the Past-40 Mr. America. The pose, you'll notice, is the same as the photo taken by my dad when I was 15.

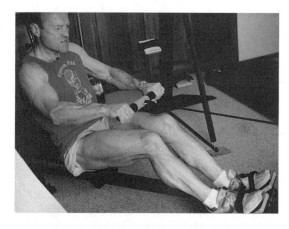

This photo taken by my wife, Carol, shows me in the throes of making a personal record for 2500 meters on the rower for submission to the Concept 2 World Rankings. My time put me in the top 25% for my age and weight.

Branching out into activities requiring both strength and stamina, I entered age-group competition on the Concept 2 Rower, where I competed at distances from 500 meters to 2500 meters. My lifetime of strength training helped most at the shorter distances. I eventually placed in the top five worldwide at 500 meters for lightweight men age 60-69.

I have also found great satisfaction in training to perform well in fitness tests at the Cooper Clinic in Dallas, Texas, the world

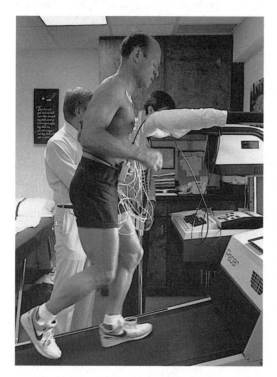

Dr. Arnie Jensen, partially shown monitoring my vital signs in the background, introduced me to the dreaded Cooper Clinic treadmill test. This photo was taken during my second visit, in 1989, where I posted a PR time of 29 minutes. *Photo by Justin Joseph*

leader in preventive medicine. Evaluations there, beginning in 1988 and continuing to the present, have placed my fitness as high as the top one percent, and always in the "superior" category for men my age.

My latest efforts have been directed toward preparing for the photos in this book. I haven't decided on my next goal, but you can bet that I will continue to pursue physical activities that challenge and excite me.

My path to success is, of course, uniquely my own. It would be a mistake for anyone else to attempt to follow in my footsteps. There's great wisdom in the maxim: "Surely the quickest path to disillusionment is the one blazed by someone else."

It's up to you to find the path that suits you best. The next section is about setting your own course—and why that's important, even crucial, for your long-term success.

The Ownership Principle Revisited

I hope you will *not* adopt the meals and exercise routines exactly as they are presented in this book, not for very long anyway. That may sound strange, because many authors would probably urge you to follow their suggestions to the letter. That might work at the beginning, but it's not likely to produce lasting results.

I would prefer that you mull over the ideas and principles presented here and select those that make sense to you, hopefully most of them, and then adapt them to suit your own preferences and circumstances.

In my book *Lean For Life*, I told about Nils Wikstrom, a Swedish health-and-fitness enthusiast who I began corresponding with in the mid-1980s. I still hear from him; we've been long-distance friends for more than 20 years. He's about my age. His letters are clearly written in perfect English and always include photos and other materials illustrating his lifestyle. Our correspondence occupies its own special place in one of our filing cabinets. I know him well. He's a classic example of the ownership principle.

He wrote to me after reading a serialized version of my first book, *Ripped*, in a British bodybuilding magazine. "I do not believe that the human body is built to lift weights for sets and repetitions as is done when bodybuilding," he wrote in that first letter. He later told me that his blood pressure went up after a year of lifting. In addition, he sent me a photo of his scar to prove that he got a hernia doing the deadlift. That experience persuaded him that the human body (or at least his body) is not built to lift heavy weights. He, however, continued to watch his diet very carefully—and eventually resumed lifting, with light weights. He also jogged around a school yard 15 minutes (no more, no less) two times per week. He cut his jog back to 5 minutes when he turned 60, but continued in a physically demanding job.

In spite of his aversion to heavy lifting, he read each of my books as they came out. He even bought a VCR especially for the purpose of watching our *Ripped* videos. In his latest letter, received a short time ago, he wrote that he never lifts more than 20-30 kilos.

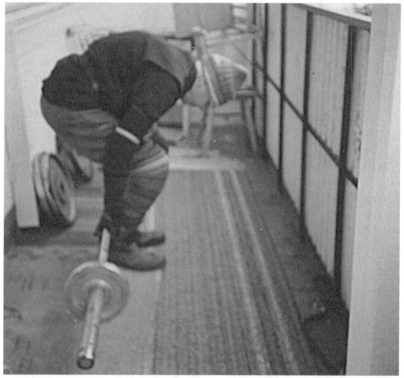

As proof, he enclosed this slightly out-of-focus photo of himself all bundled up on his balcony lifting an Olympic bar behind his legs with a 2.5 kilo plate on each side, a total of 25 kilos (55 lbs.). "I have to wear gloves as it gets too cold to hold the bar without them on," he added.

Although there doesn't seem to be anything progressive about his lifting, he obviously takes it very seriously.

To state the obvious, Nils marches to his own drummer. He doesn't follow my advice to the letter. Nevertheless, he finds value in what I have to say. He takes what he can use, and leaves the rest. That's what I suggest everyone do. Your long-term success may depend on it.

Develop your own diet and exercise program—own it—and you're more likely to stick with it.

That's what Susan Olson, Director of Psychological Services at the Southwest Geriatric Nutrition Center in Scottsdale, Arizona, and Robert Colvin of the Southern Illinois University School of Medicine, found when they studied 54 adults who had lost at least 20 percent of their body weight and had maintained the weight loss for a minimum of two years. They found plenty of variations in why and how these people succeeded. But there was one common denominator: These people each found their own method for shedding pounds and keeping them off, a method with which they were comfortable. They didn't rely on someone else's program. They developed their own.

They underwent a psychological process of "ownership." It is a process which Olson and Colvin say often spells the difference between success and failure for those trying to become lean and fit, and stay that way.

Dr. Olson says that many dieters find it much more comfortable to rely on "external" controls, such as weight-loss programs that dictate what to eat and how to act. That mind set, she says, allows the potential weight loser to feel that it's not really "up to him," that "cheating" reflects upon someone other than himself, that the control, the rules, the entire process are all out of his or her hands. Besides being untrue, such thoughts undermine a person's confidence in the suggested solution. That usually means, according to Dr. Olson, that the person soon goes back to his or her old fattening and unhealthy ways.

"It's a matter of what people are really willing and not willing to do," Dr. Olson explained. My Swedish friend Nils is not willing to lift heavy weights, but lifting 30 kilos or less and jogging around a school yard for a few minutes twice a week—and a diet with plenty of vegetables and fruit suit him just fine. That's why the routine works for him. He made the rules, and he alone is responsible for the results. It's his program. He owns it.

What's important is not the absolute correctness of his regimen, but that it makes sense to him, that he believes in it. Remember, this is his program. He developed it. It works for him. That motivates him.

Take it from my wonderful Swedish friend, if you want to stay motivated for a lifetime, develop your own health and fitness program. Own it.

Now, let's look at another author's formula for life-altering change. Unfortunately, some people refuse to change or have a very difficult time changing.

Formula for Change

Change or die! If you were given that choice, for real, could you change? Alan Deutschman asks that question in his book *Change or Die* (Regan, 2007). Unbelievable as it seems, he says the odds are nine-to-one that you would not change. He gives facts and figures to back up his assertion—and then lays out a three-part formula for beating the odds. He calls it the 3 Rs: "Relate, Repeat, and Reframe." In plain terms: "New Hope, New Skills, and New Thinking."

Deutschman gives many excellent examples, but the two that interest me most involve heart disease and his own struggle with obesity. The distressing odds he cites ring true in both cases. It is well known that the vast majority of people who lose weight gain it all back, and usually more. Weight loss, of course, is rarely a life-or-death situation. Heart disease, however, is another story. Deutschman says patients will not change their lifestyle after coronary bypass or angioplasty surgery—even if they know their life depends on it. Citing Edward Miller, MD, dean of the medical school and chief executive officer of the hospital at Johns Hopkins University as his authority, Deutschman explains that such surgeries "are no more than temporary fixes." They relieve the patient's pain, but only for a while.

Doctors tell their patients that they must "switch to a healthier lifestyle" if they want to keep the pain from coming back, avoid repeat surgery, and stop the disease before it kills them. Nevertheless, few change.

"If you look at people after coronary bypass grafting two years later, ninety percent of them have not changed their lifestyle," says Dr. Miller. "Even though they know they have a very bad disease and they know they should change their lifestyle, for whatever reason they can't."

"Facts and fear," no matter how soundly based, usually don't work. "The real key is to give people hope, not facts," says Deutschman. There's more to it, of course, but that's the crucial first step. Dr. Dean Ornish's program for heart disease sufferers is an inspiring example. You'll have to read Deutschman's book to get all the details, but here's a thumbnail sketch.

The Team Approach

Unfortunately, doctors know from their own clinical experience and research literature that the history on patient compliance is very poor. "After performing the miracle surgeries and prescribing the miracle drugs," Deutschman writes, "the doctors remind you [that] you've got to start living in a healthier way," but "they really don't believe you can change....Their lack of conviction, betrayed by the look in their eyes or the tone of their voice or their body language, takes away from the impact of their words."

What distinguishes Dean Ornish, MD, a professor of medicine at the University of California at San Francisco, is that he believes in lifestyle change—and has real-life experience and research to back it up.

After a series of smaller (and successful) trials, Ornish and his colleagues, in 1993, persuaded 194 of 333 patients with "severely clogged arteries," who had qualified for bypass or angioplasty, to forego surgery (which would practically guaranty immediate relief) and try lifestyle change instead.

"Staffers helped them quit smoking and switch to an extreme vegetarian diet that derived fewer than 10 percent of its calories from fat," Deutschman relates. "The patients got together for group conversation twice a week, and they also took classes in meditation, relaxation, yoga, and aerobic exercise, which became part of their daily routine."

After one year, when the program ended and they were on their own, one would expect them to lapse into an unhealthy lifestyle. "But three years from the start," Deutschman writes, "77 percent of the patients had stuck with these lifestyle changes—and safely avoided the need for heart surgery. They had halted—or, in many cases, reversed—the progress of their disease."

What allowed the Ornish team to reverse the odds?

Briefly, Dr. Ornish's team took the time to sell the patients on the idea that they could change; they gave them hope and made them believe in themselves. Next, they helped them learn and practice new habits and skills. Finally, they encouraged the patients to think about their disease in a new way, and to help themselves.

The Ornish approach used a team of professionals, including a cardiologist, psychologist, personal trainer, chef, and a yoga or meditation instructor, who all "fervently believe patients can change."

The approach also offered another powerful motivator: dramatic results. In all of the Ornish trials (Deutschman describes four), the frequency of chest pains fell by 90 percent or more within the first month. "The rapid improvement helps to *sell* the patients on the program and inspire them to stick with it even though it's a very demanding change," Deutschman explains.

Motivated by dramatic early success and a full year of practice (exercise, yoga or meditation, support group, and meal preparation) under the watchful eyes of the team of professionals, the patients are instilled with the understanding *and belief* necessary to continue on their own.

The bottom-line is that you've got to understand what you're doing and believe it will work. Otherwise, you're not likely to keep doing it. Makes sense, doesn't it? Why would you keep doing something you don't understand or believe?

This, of course, applies to any program of lifestyle change—including the one described and documented in this book. As explained earlier, the plan that's most likely to work is one you understand and "own."

Let's move on to the second example: the author's weight problem. We'll focus mainly on the first part of his formula, *relate* or *new hope*, because, as I see it, that's the most important obstacle to lasting change.

Hope and Obesity

At 31, Deutschman weighed 222 and was so fat that his editors at *Gentlemen's Quarterly* recruited the chief personal trainer at an upscale gym to help him lose weight. The personal trainer was a former Mr. America, which turned out to be a problem. "[He] was entirely amiable, but I could never see him as a role model," Deutschman relates. "No matter what I did, or how hard I tried, I knew that I would never look anything like him or be like him."

What's more, he says, "the place was filled with beautiful people—I was much too self-conscious and felt out of place."

He lost about six pounds at the start, but gained it all back, and soon gained six more—"which brought up my weight to its all-time peak of 228."

At 33, he moved to another city. "I was nearly resigned to the idea that I was an obese person and I simply wasn't going to change. It was becoming my identity."

Happily, that was his low point. Prodded by his girl friend, he "joined a small, friendly gym." The membership entitled him to two free sessions with one of their personal trainers. That's when things started to look up. The new trainer, an energetic young woman with "an infectious enthusiasm for exercise," turned out to be the key to solving his weight problem.

"I bonded with Claudia partly because of our similar backgrounds and interests and partly because I was intrigued by our differences," Deutschman writes. "Unlike 'Mr. America,' Claudia wasn't from another planet—she was from my planet, which made a big difference. She was like me in so many ways that it made me believe that I could be like her in the other ways—that maybe I could become fit and vibrantly healthy."

He could relate to her; she gave him hope.

Within months, his weight dropped to 188, and has stayed there for five years and counting. "I went from dreading the idea of running a one-quarter mile lap around the track to looking forward to going out and running three miles on my own."

More important than the actual process of losing weight and becoming fit (which, of course, is important), Deutschman explains, is "having a relationship with people who believe in you and whom you believe in as well... One of Claudia's great gifts is that she truly believes and expects that her clients will learn to love exercise, even if they haven't worked out much in their past."

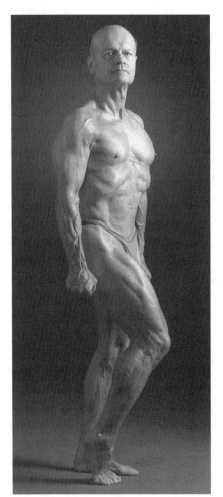

Her belief helps her clients to believe in themselves.

That's the key. You must believe in yourself and what you're doing.

My Own Case

In my own case, I believe that's why many people relate to me now who didn't relate to me when I first appeared in *Muscle & Fitness* in the early '80s. I was younger and lean, but not young enough to appeal to guys in their 20s. But now that I'm older—and still lean—and they're in their 40s, it's another story entirely. They identify with

I didn't draw the attention of the 20-something crowd in the '80s, but when they see me looking like this at 70 (and they're 40 or 50)—it inspires real hope. *Photo by Pat Berrett*

145

me now—and relate to my message. They can see themselves benefiting from my methods and example, and perhaps, in their own way, following in my footsteps.

"When you find the right relationship," Alan Deutschman proclaims, "anything is possible."

Remember, *relate* (believe), *repeat* (practice), *and reframe* (think anew). Understand what you're doing, believe in it—and live it.

You'll find many more details and examples, in medicine, science and business, in Alan Deutschman's book *Change or Die*. I urge you to read it.

My friend Dan Sawyer, who, you'll remember, told me about the new hip-replacement procedure, is a splendid example of the things we've been talking about in this chapter. I'll tell you a little more about Dan and then let him speak for himself.

DAN SAWYER: On the Shoulders of Giants

The first letter in my file from Dan is dated August 18, 1992; he refers to an earlier exchange, but we've been corresponding for at least that long. He had already read five of my books, so he was a little ahead of me in the information exchange. My file on Dan has grown very thick, but he revealed a lot about himself in that first letter.

Dan, who is older than me (he doesn't like to tell people his age, because he's afraid they will expect him to act his age, which he adamantly refuses to do) said he had "been into training and nutrition since I was in my early 20s."

Regarding his age, he wrote, "I can't help the numbers, but I can negotiate the aging process."

He had been corresponding with John Grimek, the only man to win the Mr. America contest twice and probably the most revered bodybuilder of all time. He later sent me a copy of his first letter from Grimek, dated April 14, 1975. Grimek promised him a copy of his famous pedestal pose—believed by many to be the greatest physique photo of all time. Grimek added these words of encouragement: "Glad to know you are still training. Just remember... one is NEVER too old, and exercise can be beneficial regardless of age." (And that was written more than 30 years ago!)

Dan continued: "I won't be Grimek, but I am going to be better for trying—I plug away just as if I am going to make it. This type of chasing rainbows gives me zest for living. I may get older—but never old."

I didn't know it at the time, but John Grimek is only one of many heroes/role models Dan has sought out over the years to emulate and from whom to draw strength and motivation. Dan *changed* as a young man and has striven mightily ever since to be all he can be—in many ways. I'll let him tell you about it in his own words.

As a prelude, here's a portion of what Dan wrote for our website and *Iron Game History* on the occasion of Grimek's passing in 1998:

"We are all hero oriented. Everyone carries in his mind the image of an ideal and when he sees that person he knows who it is. In my early teens John Grimek represented what I wanted to be. I told him once, 'I worked hard enough to have been a John Grimek over and over.' Compared to him I was like a candle at high noon, but I am ten thousand times better for trying. In the process I developed a lifelong quest to become better in every way and there are hundreds more who are better men because he lived."

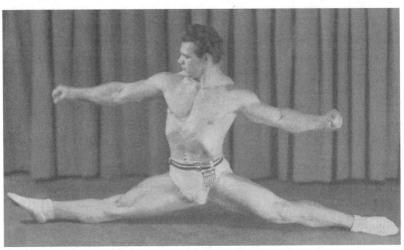

John C. Grimek, 1910–1998
Photo taken from Weight Training in Athletics (Prentice-Hall, 1956)

I asked Dan to share his philosophy on heroes, life, and aging with my readers. This is what he wrote:

> This portion of my story began somewhere in my thirteenth year. I was fairly tall and lean. I used heavy objects in the back yard to develop muscle. My father recommended I join the YMCA; I did, and my life has not been the same since.

It seems to have been a pattern. I was always attracted to people of outstanding quality. I attached myself to them and tried to be more like them. The fellow across the street was my first hero. He was handsome, outstanding physique, a fine S.A.A.U. lifter, a boxer, a perfect gentleman, and in the upper one-third of his class in medical school.

About this time, I met my second hero. He was a new English teacher who conducted a college course in high school. As a wrestler he missed the Olympics by one spot, won the Pan American Games, a gymnast, a natural athlete, and would have taught at Harvard had he not bought into the family estate. He collected rare books. The State of Louisiana built an imposing library on the Louisiana State University, Shreveport campus to house about 200,000 books he donated. He not only taught me the beauty of the written and spoken word but the YMCA triangle: *mind, body and spirit*. He impressed the value of these on me, not literally, but such that I must spend a little time each day attending to them to earn the right to do other things. He said there are twenty four hours in the day: eight to sleep, eight to work, and eight for personal attainment, meaning devote some time to enhancing your mind, body, and spirit first.

About this time, Dr. Carpenter moved next door. He was a nutritionist who made an important contribution to my life and to all I can influence.

My first admonition is to choose the right heroes. Keep in mind, even if you miss the target, the higher you aim the higher you will hit. Do something beneficial for yourself each day, and don't give up, ever. Study the works of informed people and make friends with accomplished others, and you will be molded by the company you keep.

Mother Nature has been more generous to some than to others. She produced only a few Spencers, Rachmaninoffs, Will Durants, and John Grimeks, but a host of others with less native ability.

My second admonition is even though greatness, as we think of it, is not in reach, strive for perfection as if it was a reality and you will be ten thousand times better for trying. In these matters, the great John Grimek told me, "It is never too late, you are never too old, and no matter if it comes fast or slowly, stay with it and it will come."

My third admonition is to be diligent, be persistent, and never give up. Keep your goals in front of you as if life depends on it.

The rules are simple. There is a certain academic effort required, not the same as a college major. Some trainers know more about the care of their dogs than they do for themselves. Don't drink or smoke, learn to eat that which is good for you, leave off that which is bad, take supplements for insurance, adopt an exercise program suited to your capabilities, work out thoroughly and consistently, get plenty of sleep.

My last admonition is to learn the rules, follow them, be ambitious, don't get discouraged or give up, and you will live forever.

I am totally optimistic. I can do nothing about when I was born. I may become older, but I don't want to get old, sick or die. I like it here, there is a great big wonderful world out there and I plan to see it. I want perfect health with no compromise. I know I can't beat the odds, but I intend to greatly improve on them.

Get a running start early as possible and don't stop running. Don't wait for the 'right time' to get started because the right time never comes and don't forget you can negotiate your health.

* * * *

You can see why Carol and I so highly respect Dan and cherish his friendship.

We can all benefit and learn from Dan's advice and example. I've read his essay many times and never tire of it. His admonitions and final paragraphs capture the spirit of this book.

With Dan's counsel on living long and well we can all be "totally optimistic" about realizing our own *great expectations*.

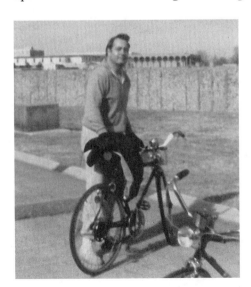

What could be more fitting than to end with a photo of Dan in his middle years; it was taken about 1983 with the L.S.U., Shreveport campus in the distant background. *Photo courtesy of Dan Sawyer*

Afterword

Author's note: *I'm sure you've noticed that most of the photos in this book were taken by Laszlo Bencze.*

Regular visitors to our website will know him for his unusual and fascinating articles about topics such as the drives and inner motivations of average lifters and strange behavior he's witnessed in gyms around the world.

Laszlo is an amazing guy. He's been lifting for more than 40 years and takes his training and that of others very seriously. He also has a lifetime of experience in photography. He takes vibrant, true-to-life, and often breathtaking family and wedding photos. He also travels the world taking photos commissioned by national and international companies; you'd recognize most of them by name. Recent assignments have taken him to China, India, Hong Kong, Germany, Austria, England, Mexico, and the Dominican Republic.

We knew he would be the perfect photographer for this book. We were also pretty sure we couldn't afford him. We were right; we couldn't. But he came anyway.

Laszlo lived with us for a full week and took more than 1400 images of just about every aspect of our lifestyle. What he did for us is priceless. Using his unique combination of lifting and fitness savvy and photographic expertise, he took photos which go beyond anything in our previous books. He captured Clarence in a different style than he has been photographed before, giving this book an exciting new look and feel, a warmer and more inviting appeal.

We asked Laszlo to give his perspective on the time he spent with us.

My Week with Basses

by Laszlo Bencze

I felt right at home with Clarence and Carol immediately. I suppose that shouldn't have surprised me given that we agree upon just about everything from training methods to movies, TV, and politics. But for me the biggest kick was actually sharing life with people who live fitness and understand it forwards and backwards. Normally I'm always explaining or making excuses for my interest in weights and muscles. In the Bass household no excuses are necessary. Here's a good example. On the day we went to Pat Berrett's studio for Clarence's official physique shots, I commented, "Hey Clarence you've got great serratus detail." And I was understood. Imagine! No blank stare. No embarrassment. This esoteric anatomical observation was just another commonplace of life. Clarence thanked me and Carol chimed in that his obliques were pretty good, too. And we're all grown ups over sixty and have raised children and owned houses. I loved it.

I will admit that they both perceived me as a fairly exotic visitor. I'm passionate about the arts, especially the visual ones and pushed Clarence into visiting several art galleries in Santa Fe which I doubt he ever would have bothered with on his own. I'm not even sure Carol could have persuaded him. (She is a devotee of the arts.) But with our combined forces, not only did he go but he actually enjoyed the experience. I have a picture of him staring at some abstractions that makes him look like an art critic.

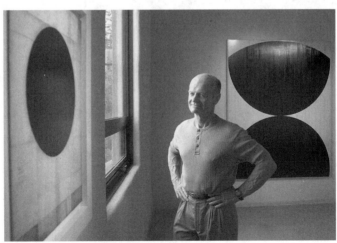

Photo by Laszlo Bencze

Of course we also hit Carl Miller's famous gym. Carl's philosophy of training centers on athletic movement as accomplished with the two Olympic lifts, the snatch and clean and jerk. He actually has novices and eighty-year-olds performing versions of these. As an old Olympic lifter myself, I think he's right on track. Nothing better develops speed and coordination than these two classic lifts. Plus, when done correctly, they are very satisfying in their own right. The trick is in doing them right and Carl is a master at coaching good performance out of even the most unlikely candidates. After all, he was once coach of the United States Olympic weightlifting team.

At the risk of presenting myself as a self-absorbed egotist, I will say that I got some admiring comments from both Clarence and Carl for doing heavy "good mornings." This is an old exercise that you never see anyone do in standard gyms because it's hard and can be dangerous. You put a barbell on your shoulders, step back from the rack, and lean forward in a deep bow. Naturally to do this without tipping forward and falling on your face you have to move your butt backwards keeping the center of gravity over your feet. It puts a ton of stress on the spinal muscles which is the point. Anyway I worked up to a set of eight with 245 pounds which I guess was jaw-dropping heavy by local standards. [By any standards]

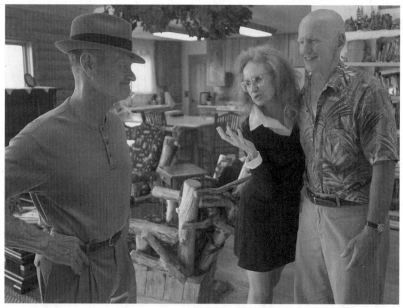

Laszlo captures Carol and Carl Miller joking with Clarence.

We all ate lunch together afterwards and it was a joy to see Clarence and Carl come alive with jokes and stories and reminiscences. These two men have been deeply involved in weight lifting and bodybuilding since they competed against each other as teenagers.

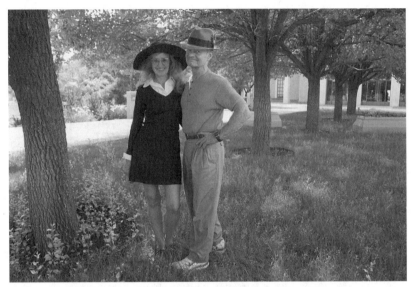

Photo by Laszlo Bencze

We said good-bye and left for the hour drive back to Albuquerque. Clarence hates to travel. He's a genuine home body. So I was amused to observe his concern about "finding the road back to Albuquerque" as if we were in the Amazon basin and not sure of our tributary. Goodness, there's only one interstate between the two cities and a blind person could find it in a few minutes. But hey, we all have our little idiosyncrasies. As the Basses found out, one of mine is meticulously clean windshields. I had to scrub the glass on both their cars inside and out before I was satisfied.

Now I ought to talk a bit about dieting. There is nothing Clarence has emphasized more than the need to forget about "dieting" and to develop an eating style. I've read his books and thought I understood this principle, but there's no substitute for first hand experience. And that's what made me realize I really hadn't understood it until I experienced it.

When Clarence says you shouldn't feel deprived by your diet, *he really means it*! The breakfasts he served me during the week were huge. Several times I came close to not being able to finish and I'm a big eater. I had to force myself to keep eating the mixture of grains, vegetables, fruits, and ground flaxseed accompanied by a glass of soy milk. I can assure you when I left the table there was no residual hunger. I was stuffed. And that's the point. I was stuffed with low caloric bulky food which actually tasted good.

By the way, one of Clarence's principles for tricking yourself into thinking you're eating a lot (as if you needed any such trickery) is to use a teaspoon instead of a tablespoon to eat your cereal. I joked that he ought to design a new and improved teaspoon specifically for dieting, call it the "Clarence Bass Dietetic Spoon," and market it for $39.95. Sadly, this will never happen. He's a strict no-gimmicks kind of guy.

Secondly, you score no points with Clarence by skipping snacks. He won't pat you on the head and call you a good boy for not having that mid-morning Tiger's Milk bar and apple. Instead he'll tell you you're missing the point. The snacks are there to keep your blood sugar at a steady level and to keep you from developing the pangs that will cause you to stuff yourself at your next meal. Does the principal work? You bet it does. When lunch rolled around, I was ready to eat but found I was satisfied with a much smaller meal than I would have taken in the past.

The mid-afternoon snack came in handy. It helped fuel me through a couple of workouts that went much more smoothly than in the past when I would eat nothing between lunch and dinner. Sure I could get through my workouts pretty well without eating the snack. If you really want to you can push yourself to do unpleasant things and you can do them regularly. But trust me; it was so much more pleasant doing the workout with a snack in my belly. I could push even harder. (Maybe that's one reason my good morning workout went so impressively.)

Dinner with the Basses always starts with a gargantuan salad. I mean by this enough for two badgers or four rabbits. Carol sprinkles a couple tablespoons of balsamic vinegar and one of olive oil over the greens, tomatoes, avocados, celery, romaine lettuce, green beans, and whatever else catches her fancy at the market. Frankly, I've never been much of a salad fan. Perhaps this is because so many restaurant salads are so boring with their pathetic shaved carrot on top of some iceberg lettuce that looks like it had melted. The principle is it doesn't much matter what you throw in your salad as long as it's fresh, tasty, and bulky. And don't lard on the dressing. The balsamic vinegar is just right to give it all a savory flavor. (Don't buy the cheap stuff like I did. It'll burn your mouth and make you think you're eating something from a chemistry set. Go for the expensive, aged, balsamic. It makes all the difference.)

The main meal can be chicken, fish, beans, or anything that's not swimming in cheese sauce and cream. I'm no expert on cooking so you'll have to go elsewhere for that info. But apparently there are lots of books telling you how to cook healthy low-fat entrees.

Finally comes the evening snack. This is two slices of bread with a dollop of peanut or almond butter, and a bit of fruit preserve. This is tasty, textured, satisfying, and not particularly high in calories, especially compared with eating a pint of ice cream or bag of potato chips. Again the focus is on bulk and pleasure. Clarence cuts his peanut butter sandwich into four pieces and consumes one per quarter hour as he watches TV. (I'm not making this up.) I gave it a try myself and found that I could match him quarter sandwich per quarter hour and even outlast him by a few seconds.

There you go. Lots of food. No deprivation. No weighing things or counting calories. It's exactly what Clarence says: an eating style. I'm continuing to do it myself here at home and I can tell it's working. I'm eating less than I used to and slowly, very slowly losing weight. Clarence suggested going down an average of half a pound a week to reach my target weight of 225. Starting from 252, that should take about a year which is just right. Slow weight loss doesn't upset the body and push it into the starvation response which changes metabolism and packs on flab.

Clarence had not invited me just to be a house guest. I had a job to do. I had to take pictures that would meet his expectations of showing how an older man can be a first rate bodybuilder yet still have a normal, non-obsessive lifestyle. He wanted pictures taken at home, walking around the neighborhood, visiting with friends, as well as exercising. Fortunately, I found that I could persuade Clarence to pose just about anytime I wanted him to, in ways he had never before considered. This was fun. The results are scattered throughout this book and I hope you readers have enjoyed them.

21 Jul. '07

Laszlo Bencze
360-896-2637
commercial: www.lbencze.com
weddings: www.laszlophoto.com
laszlo@lbencze.com

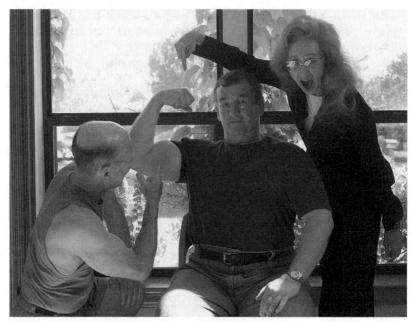

Wow! Laszlo has a humongous biceps; pretty good for a guy who doesn't consider himself a bodybuilder.

Postscript

About My Other Books

All of my books are different. *Great Expectations* is my ninth book. It presents my perspective at 70, after more than 55 years of training. My outlook and aspirations at 42, when my first book, *RIPPED* came out, were different. The same is true of *Lean For Life*, written when I was 52, and *Challenge Yourself*, at 61. All of my books cover new ground. Each book builds on the earlier books—but does not replace them.

It may surprise you to know that *RIPPED: The Sensible Way to Achieve Ultimate Muscularity* is still one of our best sellers. Now in its eleventh printing, *RIPPED* is the story of my first confirmed reduction to 2.4% body fat, and my wins at the Past-40 Mr. America and USA contests. It tells how my study of sensible fat loss began. I recount my many underwater weighings at the famous Lovelace Medical Center (known for its testing of the original astronauts) and explain the critical role body composition tests played in shaping my philosophy of diet and exercise. What distinguishes *RIPPED* from perhaps any other book of its kind is the focus on my thinking process, revealing the mistakes I made as well as what I did right, and how both contributed to my success. That's significant because it's the same trial-and-error process you will go through to solve your own weight and muscle building problems. Almost none of that is in this book or my other books. *RIPPED* provides the platform or springboard for the books that follow.

Many say they benefited from all eight of my previous books. I grew and learned with each one and like to think my readers do as well. Some or all of my books might help you achieve current or future goals. I'll tell you a little about each one and you can decide.

The three-book *RIPPED* series is for bodybuilders and others interested in developing ultimate muscularity using healthy means. As indicated above, *RIPPED* is about a trial-and-error learning process. *RIPPED 2* has been called the best book ever written on training; it includes an in-depth exploration of hard/easy exercise, the all-or-none principle of muscle fiber contraction, the meaning of intensity, coping with calories, the famine phenomenon, navigating the last few weeks before competition, and training psychology. *RIPPED 3: The Recipes, The Routines & The Reasons* is just what the sub-title says. It includes 22 meal plans and comments designed to help readers plan and prepare their own recipes to make and keep them lean. Building on the hard/easy method described in *RIPPED 2*, the third book explains and lays out the first bodybuilding routines using periodization. Finally, it explains the problem with aerobics for bodybuilders and suggests a solution to obtain the fat-burning benefits of aerobic exercise without sacrificing hard-earned muscle tissue.

Lean For Life is for those interested in becoming and staying lean and fit, but not necessarily champion bodybuilders or competitive athletes. It details both the *how* and *why* of healthy eating and exercising. It tells day-by-day how to combine weights and aerobics to achieve total fitness. Motivation is one of the main themes; it explains how to stay motivated for the long-term. The final chapter introduces the "Ownership Principle," which is revisited in this book. *Lean For Life* presents a well-rounded lifestyle approach to make and keep you lean forever.

It's easy to confuse *Lean For Life* and *The Lean Advantage* series because the similar titles. *The Lean Advantage 1, 2, and 3* are a collection of 155 columns I wrote for *Muscle & Fitness* magazine from 1980 to 1994. The format is mostly question and answer, and the subjects covered include just about everything relating to fitness, health, and fat loss. Topics are organized under 12 to 16 chapter headings, depending on the volume. Taken together, the three books constitute a virtual encyclopedia of the bodybuilding and fitness lifestyle. Many of the topics are not covered in my other books.

Challenge Yourself is my last book before this one. As suggested by the title, the theme is challenge; it says the key to becoming—and staying—lean, fit, and healthy is to continually challenge yourself to improve in an intelligent and thoughtful way. For the first time, I discuss the importance of "good" fat and give model meals containing healthy fats. I also explain the Glycemic Index and how to use it most effectively. I compare and contrast the volume and high-intensity approaches to training, and introduce an entry-level mass and strength routine combining the two methods. *Challenge Yourself* talks about the advantages of athletic-type lifting and gives newly discovered information on the benefits of high-intensity aerobics; it also outlines my personal routine utilizing both concepts. Finally, it includes a chapter on longevity and health issues, and ends with inspiring profiles of older athletes who thrive on challenge.

Finally, I want to tell you about our DVDs. I have written and produced, in cooperation with our Australian friends Wayne and Tina Gallasch, three DVDs designed to complement my books. They demonstrate things that are difficult to explain adequately in a book. *Ripped The DVD* includes preparation of my "Old Reliable" breakfast, use of a training diary, athletic-type lifting, high-intensity aerobics, lower ab and oblique training, post-workout meal, bedtime snack, and tracking changes in body fat—plus a short posing segment. The *Second RIPPED DVD* takes up where the first leaves off, adding a whole-body weight workout, interval workouts on the treadmill and rower, behind-the-scenes at a studio photo shoot, along with a series of conversations explaining core concepts and introducing the action segments.

Completely different, *The Third RIPPED DVD* uses real life stories to illustrate motivation builders and killers. Wayne, Tina, and I tell revealing stories about ourselves. Wayne's story is about competition, the ultimate motivator. He relates how he transformed himself from a fitness buff, lifting weights in his basement, to the world's best 500-meter indoor rower for his age and weight. I explain the mastery approach and how trying to keep up with Wayne almost sidelined me. Tina's story may be the best of all. She tells about discovering, to her great surprise, that she enjoyed indoor rowing and lifting, and how the revelation converted her from a couch potato to an avid trainer.

If *Great Expectations* is the first of my books you've read, I hope I have persuaded you that it should not be your last.

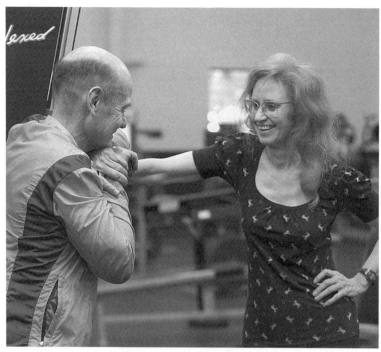

Photo by Laszlo Bencze

My Wife, the Enabler

My wife Carol means everything to me. I couldn't live without her—not in the way I live now. She is an enabler, in the best sense of the word, because she does the things that I can't or won't do, so I can focus on doing what I do best.

I'm a good writer, but she makes me a better writer. I resist mightily when she tells me I didn't explain something well enough or that I'm bogging readers down with too much detail. I've learned, however, that her lifetime love of reading has given her a keen sense of what readers want and need. She's almost always right. So I eventually settle down and do my best to fix the problem.

I hope you will join me in thanking her for putting up with me—and making this book much better than I could make it on my own. She turned a rocky creek into a flowing stream.